Skills Checklist to Accompany

FUNDAMENTALS OF NURSING

STANDARDS & PRACTICE

THIRD EDITION

Sue C. DeLaune, MN, RN
Assistant Professor
School of Nursing
William Carey College
New Orleans, Louisiana

President and Educational Director
SDeLaune Consulting
Mandeville, Louisiana

Patricia K. Ladner MS, MN, RN
Consultant for Nursing Practice
Louisiana State Board of Nursing
New Orleans, Louisiana

Prepared by
Julie Sanford, DNS, RN
Assistant Professor
California State University in San Bernardino
San Bernardino, California

THOMSON

DELMAR LEARNING

Australia Canada Mexico Singapore Spain United Kingdom United States

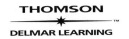

THOMSON

DELMAR LEARNING

**Skills Checklist to Accompany Fundamentals of Nursing: Standards and Practice
Third Edition**

By Sue C. DeLaune and Patricia K. Ladner
Prepared by Julie Sanford DNS, RN

Vice President, Health Care Business Unit:
William Brottmiller

Editorial Director:
Matthew Kane

Acquisitions Editor:
Tamara Caruso

Developmental Editor:
Patricia A. Gaworecki

Marketing Director:
Jennifer McAvey

Marketing Coordinator:
Michele McTighe

Editorial Assistant:
Tiffiny Adams

Production Director:
Carolyn S. Miller

Production Coordinator:
Mary Ellen Cox

Senior Project Editor:
David Buddle

Art and Design Specialist:
Robert Plante

Library of Congress Catalog Number:
2005028584

ISBN 10: 1-4018-5920-8
ISBN 13: 978-1-4018-5920-8

Contents

Procedure 26-1:	Measuring Body Temperature	1
Procedure 26-2:	Assessing Pulse Rate	9
Procedure 26-3:	Assessing Respiration	13
Procedure 26-4:	Assessing Blood Pressure	15
Procedure 28-1:	Performing Venipuncture (Blood Drawing)	19
Procedure 28-2:	Performing a Skin Puncture	25
Procedure 28-3:	Obtaining a Residual Urine Specimen from an Indwelling Catheter	29
Procedure 28-4:	Collecting a Clean-Catch, Midstream Urine Specimen	31
Procedure 28-5:	Measuring Blood Glucose Levels	35
Procedure 29-1:	Applying Restraints	39
Procedure 29-2:	Handwashing	43
Procedure 29-3:	Applying Sterile Gloves via the Open Method	45
Procedure 29-4:	Donning and Removing Clean and Contaminated Gloves, Cap, and Mask	49
Procedure 29-5:	Surgical Hand Antisepsis	53
Procedure 29-6:	Applying Sterile Gloves and Gown via the Closed Method	57
Procedure 29-7:	Removing Contaminated Items	59
Procedure 29-8:	Bathing a Client in Bed	63
Procedure 29-9:	Changing Linens in an Unoccupied Bed	67
Procedure 29-10:	Changing Linens in an Occupied Bed	73
Procedure 29-11:	Perineal and Genital Care	77
Procedure 29-12:	Oral Care	79
Procedure 29-13:	Eye Care	87
Procedure 30-1:	Medication Administration: Oral, Sublingual, and Buccal	95
Procedure 30-2:	Withdrawing Medication from an Ampule	99
Procedure 30-3:	Withdrawing Medication from a Vial	101
Procedure 30-4:	Mixing Medications from Two Vials into One Syringe	103
Procedure 30-5:	Medication Administration: Intradermal	107
Procedure 30-6:	Medication Administration: Subcutaneous	109
Procedure 30-7:	Medication Administration: Intramuscular	111
Procedure 30-8:	Medication Administration: Secondary Administration Sets (Piggyback)	113
Procedure 30-9:	Medication Administration: Eye and Ear	115
Procedure 30-10:	Medication Administration: Nasal	121
Procedure 30-11:	Medication Administration: Nebulizer	123
Procedure 30-12:	Medication Administration: Rectal	129
Procedure 30-13:	Medication Administration: Vaginal	133
Procedure 31-1:	Administering Therapeutic Massage	137
Procedure 32-1:	Maintaining and Cleaning the Tracheostomy Tube	141
Procedure 32-2:	Performing Nasopharyngeal and Oropharyngeal Suctioning	147
Procedure 32-3:	Suctioning Endotracheal and Tracheal Tubes	153

Procedure 32-4:	Administering Oxygen Therapy	157
Procedure 32-5:	Performing the Heimlich Maneuver	153
Procedure 32-6:	Administering Cardiopulmonary Resuscitation (CPR)	169
Procedure 33-1:	Measuring Intake and Output	177
Procedure 33-2:	Preparing an IV Solution	179
Procedure 33-3:	Preparing the IV Bag and Tubing	183
Procedure 33-4:	Assessing and Maintaining an IV Insertion Site	185
Procedure 33-5:	Changing the IV Solution	187
Procedure 33-6:	Flushing a Central Venous Catheter	189
Procedure 33-7:	Setting the IV Flow Rate	191
Procedure 33-8:	Changing the Central Venous Dressing	193
Procedure 33-9:	Discontinuing the IV and Changing to a Saline or Heparin Lock	195
Procedure 33-10:	Administering a Blood Transfusion	199
Procedure 34-1:	Inserting a Nasogastric or Nasointestinal Tube for Suction and Enteral Feedings	203
Procedure 34-2:	Administering Enteral Tube Feedings	209
Procedure 35-1:	Administering Patient-Controlled Analgesia (PCA)	215
Procedure 35-2:	Administering Epidural Analgesia	219
Procedure 36-1:	Proper Body Mechanics, Safe Lifting, and Transferring	223
Procedure 36-2:	Administering Passive Range of Motion (ROM) Exercises	227
Procedure 36-3:	Turning and Positioning a Client	233
Procedure 36-4:	Moving a Client in Bed	239
Procedure 36-5:	Assisting from Bed to Wheelchair, Commode, or Chair	245
Procedure 36-6:	Assisting from Bed to Stretcher	249
Procedure 36-7:	Using a Hydraulic Lift	253
Procedure 36-8:	Assisting with Ambulation and Safe Walking	257
Procedure 36-9:	Assisting with Crutches, Cane, or Walker	261
Procedure 37-1:	Obtaining a Wound Drainage Specimen for Culturing	269
Procedure 37-2:	Irrigating a Wound	271
Procedure 37-3:	Applying a Dry Dressing	275
Procedure 37-4:	Applying a Wet to Damp Dressing (Wet to Moist Dressing)	279
Procedure 37-5:	Preventing and Managing the Pressure Ulcer	283
Procedure 39-1:	Assisting with a Bedpan or Urinal	287
Procedure 39-2:	Applying a Condom Catheter	291
Procedure 39-3:	Inserting an Indwelling Catheter: Male	295
Procedure 39-4:	Inserting an Indwelling Catheter: Female	301
Procedure 39-5:	Irrigating an Open Urinary Catheter	307
Procedure 39-6:	Irrigating the Bladder Using a Closed-System Catheter	311
Procedure 39-7:	Administering an Enema	317
Procedure 39-8:	Irrigating and Cleaning a Stoma	325
Procedure 40-1:	Postoperative Exercise Instruction	329
Procedure 40-2:	Pulse Oximetry	333

Preface

The skills checklists in this manual are summaries of the step-by-step procedures in *Fundamentals of Nursing: Standards & Practice,* third edition, by Sue DeLaune and Pat Ladner. Each checklist matches the procedure as described in the textbook.

To use the skills checklists most effectively, the student should refer to the procedure first, then "practice," referring to the checklist. Some procedures have segments that may not be used at once. These segments are bolded so students can focus on/perform certain parts of the procedures.

When students are evaluated using the checklists, there are three categories to document their performances of the skills: "Able to Perform," "Able to Perform with Assistance," and "Unable to Perform." These categories lend themselves to the college laboratory setting as well as to the clinical setting, where students may perform procedures with faculty assistance.

Procedures in Textbook

The accompanying procedures for the checklists can be found on the following pages in *Fundamentals of Nursing Standards & Practice*, third edition.

Chapter 26
Procedure 26-1: Measuring Body Temperature — 1
Procedure 26-2: Assessing Pulse Rate — 9
Procedure 26-3: Assessing Respiration — 13
Procedure 26-4: Assessing Blood Pressure — 15

Chapter 28
Procedure 28-1: Performing Venipuncture (Blood Drawing) — 19
Procedure 28-2: Performing a Skin Puncture — 25
Procedure 28-3: Obtaining a Residual Urine Specimen from an Indwelling Catheter — 29
Procedure 28-4: Collecting a Clean-Catch, Midstream Urine Specimen — 31
Procedure 28-5: Measuring Blood Glucose Levels — 35

Chapter 29
Procedure 29-1: Applying Restraints — 39
Procedure 29-2: Handwashing — 43
Procedure 29-3: Applying Sterile Gloves via the Open Method — 45
Procedure 29-4: Donning and Removing Clean and Contaminated Gloves, Cap, and Mask — 49
Procedure 29-5: Surgical Hand Antisepsis — 53
Procedure 29-6: Applying Sterile Gloves and Gown via the Closed Method — 57
Procedure 29-7: Removing Contaminated Items — 59
Procedure 29-8: Bathing a Client in Bed — 63
Procedure 29-9: Changing Linens in an Unoccupied Bed — 67
Procedure 29-10: Changing Linens in an Occupied Bed — 73
Procedure 29-11: Perineal and Genital Care — 77
Procedure 29-12: Oral Care — 79
Procedure 29-13: Eye Care — 87

Chapter 30
Procedure 30-1: Medication Administration: Oral, Sublingual, and Buccal — 95
Procedure 30-2: Withdrawing Medication from an Ampule — 99
Procedure 30-3: Withdrawing Medication from a Vial — 101
Procedure 30-4: Mixing Medications from Two Vials into One Syringe — 103
Procedure 30-5: Medication Administration: Intradermal — 107
Procedure 30-6: Medication Administration: Subcutaneous — 109
Procedure 30-7: Medication Administration: Intramuscular — 111
Procedure 30-8: Medication Administration: Secondary Administration Sets (Piggyback) — 113

Procedure 30-9: Medication Administration: Eye and Ear — 115
Procedure 30-10: Medication Administration: Nasal — 121
Procedure 30-11: Medication Administration: Nebulizer — 123
Procedure 30-12: Medication Administration: Rectal — 129
Procedure 30-13: Medication Administration: Vaginal — 133

Chapter 31
Procedure 31-1: Administering Therapeutic Massage — 137

Chapter 32
Procedure 32-1: Maintaining and Cleaning the Tracheostomy Tube — 141
Procedure 32-2: Performing Nasopharyngeal and Oropharyngeal Suctioning — 147
Procedure 32-3: Suctioning Endotracheal and Tracheal Tubes — 153
Procedure 32-4: Administering Oxygen Therapy — 157
Procedure 32-5: Performing the Heimlich Maneuver — 163
Procedure 32-6: Administering Cardiopulmonary Resuscitation (CPR) — 169

Chapter 33
Procedure 33-1: Measuring Intake and Output — 177
Procedure 33-2: Preparing an IV Solution — 179
Procedure 33-3: Preparing the IV Bag and Tubing — 183
Procedure 33-4: Assessing and Maintaining an IV Insertion Site — 185
Procedure 33-5: Changing the IV Solution — 187
Procedure 33-6: Flushing a Central Venous Catheter — 189
Procedure 33-7: Setting the IV Flow Rate — 191
Procedure 33-8: Changing the Central Venous Dressing — 193
Procedure 33-9: Discontinuing the IV and Changing to a Saline or Heparin Lock — 195
Procedure 33-10: Administering a Blood Transfusion — 199

Chapter 34
Procedure 34-1: Inserting a Nasogastric or Nasointestinal Tube for Suction and Enteral Feedings — 203
Procedure 34-2: Administering Enteral Tube Feedings — 209

Chapter 35
Procedure 35-1: Administering Patient-Controlled Analgesia (PCA) — 215
Procedure 35-2: Administering Epidural Analgesia — 219

Chapter 36
Procedure 36-1: Proper Body Mechanics, Safe Lifting, and Transferring — 223
Procedure 36-2: Administering Passive Range-of-Motion (ROM) Exercises — 227

Procedure 36-3:   Turning and Positioning a Client   233
Procedure 36-4:   Moving a Client in Bed   239
Procedure 36-5:   Assisting from Bed to Wheelchair, Commode, or Chair   245
Procedure 36-6:   Assisting from Bed to Stretcher   249
Procedure 36-7:   Using a Hydraulic Lift   253
Procedure 36-8:   Assisting with Ambulation and Safe Walking   257
Procedure 36-9:   Assisting with Crutches, Cane, or Walker   261

Chapter 37
Procedure 37-1:   Obtaining a Wound Drainage Specimen for Culturing   269
Procedure 37-2:   Irrigating a Wound   271
Procedure 37-3:   Applying a Dry Dressing   275
Procedure 37-4:   Applying a Wet-to-Damp Dressing (Wet-to-Moist Dressing)   279
Procedure 37-5:   Preventing and Managing the Pressure Ulcer   283

Chapter 39
Procedure 39-1:   Assisting with a Bedpan or Urinal   287
Procedure 39-2:   Applying a Condom Catheter   291
Procedure 39-3:   Inserting an Indwelling Catheter: Male   295
Procedure 39-4:   Inserting an Indwelling Catheter: Female   301
Procedure 39-5:   Irrigating an Open Urinary Catheter   307
Procedure 39-6:   Irrigating the Bladder Using a Closed-System Catheter   311
Procedure 39-7:   Administering an Enema   317
Procedure 39-8:   Irrigating and Cleaning a Stoma   325

Chapter 40
Procedure 40-1:   Postoperative Exercise Instruction   329
Procedure 40-2:   Pulse Oximetry   333

Checklist for Procedure 26-1   Measuring Body Temperature

Name _____ Date _____

School _____

Instructor _____

Course _____

Procedure 26-1 Measuring Body Temperature	Able to Perform	Able to Perform with Assistance	Unable to Perform	Initials/Date
1. Review medical record for baseline factors that influence vital signs. *Comments:*	☐	☐	☐	
2. Explain to client that vital signs will be assessed. Encourage client to remain still and refrain from drinking, eating, and smoking, and to avoid mouth breathing, if possible. *Comments:*	☐	☐	☐	
3. Assess client's toileting needs and proceed as appropriate. *Comments:*	☐	☐	☐	
4. Gather equipment. *Comments:*	☐	☐	☐	
5. Provide for privacy. *Comments:*	☐	☐	☐	
6. Wash hands/hand hygiene and apply gloves, when appropriate. *Comments:*	☐	☐	☐	
Oral Temperature: Electronic Thermometer 7. Repeat Actions 1–6. *Comments:*	☐	☐	☐	

continued on the following page

continued from the previous page

Procedure 26-1 Measuring Body Temperature	Able to Perform	Able to Perform with Assistance	Unable to Perform	Initials/Date
8. Place disposable protective sheath over probe. *Comments:*	☐	☐	☐	
9. Grasp top of probe's stem. *Comments:*	☐	☐	☐	
10. Place tip of thermometer under the client's tongue and along gumline to posterior sublingual pocket lateral to center of lower jaw. *Comments:*	☐	☐	☐	
11. Instruct client to keep mouth closed around thermometer. *Comments:*	☐	☐	☐	
12. Thermometer will signal (beep) when a constant temperature registers. *Comments:*	☐	☐	☐	
13. Read measurement on digital display of electronic thermometer. Push ejection button to discard disposable sheath into receptacle and return probe to storage well. *Comments:*	☐	☐	☐	
14. Inform client of temperature reading. *Comments:*	☐	☐	☐	
15. Remove gloves and perform hand hygiene. *Comments:*	☐	☐	☐	

continued on the following page

continued from the previous page

Procedure 26-1 Measuring Body Temperature	Able to Perform	Able to Perform with Assistance	Unable to Perform	Initials/Date
16. Record reading according to institution policies. *Comments:*	☐	☐	☐	
17. Return electronic thermometer unit to charging base. *Comments:*	☐	☐	☐	
18. Wash hands/hand hygiene. *Comments:*	☐	☐	☐	
Tympanic Temperature: Infrared Thermometer 19. Repeat Actions 1–6. *Comments:*	☐	☐	☐	
20. Position client in Sims' or sitting position. *Comments:*	☐	☐	☐	
21. Remove probe from container and attach probe cover to tympanic thermometer unit. *Comments:*	☐	☐	☐	
22. Turn client's head to one side. Gently insert probe with firm pressure into ear canal. *Comments:*	☐	☐	☐	
23. Remove probe after the reading is displayed on digital unit (usually 2 seconds). *Comments:*	☐	☐	☐	

continued on the following page

continued from the previous page

Procedure 26-1 Measuring Body Temperature	Able to Perform	Able to Perform with Assistance	Unable to Perform	Initials/Date
24. Remove probe cover and replace in storage container. *Comments:*	☐	☐	☐	
25. Return tympanic thermometer to storage unit. *Comments:*	☐	☐	☐	
26. Record reading according to institution policy. *Comments:*	☐	☐	☐	
27. Hand hygiene. *Comments:*	☐	☐	☐	
Using a "Tempa-Dot" 28. Repeat Actions 1–6. *Comments:*	☐	☐	☐	
29. Position the client in a sitting or lying position. *Comments:*	☐	☐	☐	
30. Prepare Tempa-Dot according to directions. • Oral measurement: Place Tempa-Dot under tongue as far back as possible. Have client press tongue down on thermometer and keep mouth closed for 60 seconds. Remove thermometer, read the last blue dot; ignore any skipped dot.	☐	☐	☐	

continued on the following page

continued from the previous page

Procedure 26-1 Measuring Body Temperature	Able to Perform	Able to Perform with Assistance	Unable to Perform	Initials/Date
• Auxiliary measurement. Place thermometer high in the armpit, vertical to the body, with dots against the torso. Lower client's arm to hold thermometer in place. Remove thermometer after 3 minutes. *Comments:*				
31. Record temperature, indicate the method, and discard the thermometer. *Comments:*	☐	☐	☐	
32. Wash hands/hand hygiene. *Comments:*	☐	☐	☐	
33. Repeat Actions 1–6. *Comments:*	☐	☐	☐	
34. Position client in a sitting or lying position with head of the bed elevated from 45° to 60° for measurement of all vital signs except those designated otherwise. *Comments:*	☐	☐	☐	
Rectal Temperature 35. Repeat Actions 1–6. *Comments:*	☐	☐	☐	
36. Place client in the Sims' position with upper knee flexed. Adjust sheet to expose only anal area. *Comments:*	☐	☐	☐	

continued on the following page

continued from the previous page

Procedure 26-1 Measuring Body Temperature	Able to Perform	Able to Perform with Assistance	Unable to Perform	Initials/Date
37. Place tissues in easy reach. Apply gloves. *Comments:*	☐	☐	☐	
38. Lubricate rectal probe tip. *Comments:*	☐	☐	☐	
39. With dominant hand, grasp top of the probe's stem. With other hand, separate buttocks to expose anus. *Comments:*	☐	☐	☐	
40. Instruct client to take a deep breath. Insert probe gently into anus. *Comments:*	☐	☐	☐	
41. Repeat Actions 12–18. *Comments:*	☐	☐	☐	
Axillary Temperature 42. Repeat Actions 1–6. *Comments:*	☐	☐	☐	
43. Remove client's arm and shoulder from one sleeve of gown. Avoid exposing chest. *Comments:*	☐	☐	☐	
44. Make sure axillary skin is dry; if necessary, pat dry. *Comments:*	☐	☐	☐	

continued on the following page

continued from the previous page

Procedure 26-1 Measuring Body Temperature	Able to Perform	Able to Perform with Assistance	Unable to Perform	Initials/Date
45. Place probe into center of axilla. Fold client's upper arm straight down, and place arm across client's chest. *Comments:*	☐	☐	☐	
46. Repeat Actions 12–18. *Comments:*	☐	☐	☐	
Disposable (Chemical Strip) Thermometer 47. Repeat Actions 1–6. *Comments:*	☐	☐	☐	
48. Apply tape to appropriate skin area, usually forehead. *Comments:*	☐	☐	☐	
49. Observe tape for color changes. *Comments:*	☐	☐	☐	
50. Record reading and indicate method. *Comments:*	☐	☐	☐	
51. Wash hands/hand hygiene. *Comments:*	☐	☐	☐	

Checklist for Procedure 26-2   Assessing Pulse Rate

Name _____ Date _____

School _____

Instructor _____

Course _____

Procedure 26-2 Assessing Pulse Rate	Able to Perform	Able to Perform with Assistance	Unable to Perform	Initials/Date
Taking a Radial (Wrist) Pulse 1. Wash hands/hand hygiene. *Comments:*	☐	☐	☐	
2. Inform client of site(s) where pulse will be measured. *Comments:*	☐	☐	☐	
3. Flex client's elbow and place lower part of arm across chest. *Comments:*	☐	☐	☐	
4. Support client's wrist by grasping outer aspect with thumb. *Comments:*	☐	☐	☐	
5. Place index and middle fingers on inner aspect of client's wrist over the radial artery, and apply light but firm pressure until pulse is palpated. *Comments:*	☐	☐	☐	
6. Identify pulse rhythm. *Comments:*	☐	☐	☐	
7. Determine pulse volume. *Comments:*	☐	☐	☐	

continued on the following page

continued from the previous page

Procedure 26-2 Assessing Pulse Rate	Able to Perform	Able to Perform with Assistance	Unable to Perform	Initials/Date
8. Count pulse rate by using second hand on watch. *Comments:*	☐	☐	☐	
Taking an Apical Pulse 9. Wash hands/hand hygiene. *Comments:*	☐	☐	☐	
10. Raise client's gown to expose sternum and left side of chest. *Comments:*	☐	☐	☐	
11. Cleanse earpiece and stethoscope diaphragm with an alcohol swab. *Comments:*	☐	☐	☐	
12. Put stethoscope around neck. *Comments:*	☐	☐	☐	
13. Locate apex of heart. • With client lying on left side, locate suprasternal notch. • Palpate second intercostals space to left of sternum. • Place index finger in intercostals space, counting downward until fifth intercostals space is located. • Move index finger along fourth intercostals space left of sternal border and to fifth intercostals space, left of midclavicular line to palpate the point of maximal impulse (PMI). • Keep index finger of nondominant hand on PMI. *Comments:*	☐	☐	☐	

continued on the following page

continued from the previous page

Procedure 26-2 Assessing Pulse Rate	Able to Perform	Able to Perform with Assistance	Unable to Perform	Initials/Date
14. Inform client that client's heart will be listened to. Instruct client to remain silent. *Comments:*	☐	☐	☐	
15. With dominant hand, put earpiece of the stethoscope in ears and grasp diaphragm of stethoscope in palm of the hand for 5–10 seconds. *Comments:*	☐	☐	☐	
16. Place diaphragm of stethoscope over PMI and auscultate for sounds S_1 and S_2 to hear lub-dub sound. *Comments:*	☐	☐	☐	
17. Note regularity of rhythm. *Comments:*	☐	☐	☐	
18. Start to count while looking at second hand of watch. Count lub-dub sound as one beat. • For a regular rhythm, count rate for 30 seconds and multiply by 2. • For an irregular rhythm, count rate for a full minute, noting number of irregular beats. *Comments:*	☐	☐	☐	
19. Share findings with client. *Comments:*	☐	☐	☐	
20. Record by site: rate, rhythm, and, if applicable, number of irregular beats. *Comments:*	☐	☐	☐	

continued on the following page

continued from the previous page

Procedure 26-2 Assessing Pulse Rate	Able to Perform	Able to Perform with Assistance	Unable to Perform	Initials/Date
21. Wash hands/hand hygiene. *Comments:*	☐	☐	☐	

Checklist for Procedure 26-3 Assessing Respiration

Name _____ Date _____

School _____

Instructor _____

Course _____

Procedure 26-3 Assessing Respiration	Able to Perform	Able to Perform with Assistance	Unable to Perform	Initials/Date
1. Wash hands/hand hygiene. *Comments:*	☐	☐	☐	
2. Be sure chest movement is visible. Remove heavy clothing, if necessary. *Comments:*	☐	☐	☐	
3. Observe one complete respiratory cycle. *Comments:*	☐	☐	☐	
4. Start counting with first inspiration while looking at the second hand of a watch. • If an irregular rate or rhythm is present, count for 1 full minute. *Comments:*	☐	☐	☐	
5. Observe character of respiration. *Comments:*	☐	☐	☐	
6. Replace client's gown, if needed. *Comments:*	☐	☐	☐	
7. Record rate and character of respirations. *Comments:*	☐	☐	☐	
8. Wash hands/hand hygiene. *Comments:*	☐	☐	☐	

Checklist for Procedure 26-4   Assessing Blood Pressure

Name _____ Date _____

School _____

Instructor _____

Course _____

Procedure 26-4 Assessing Blood Pressure	Able to Perform	Able to Perform with Assistance	Unable to Perform	Initials/Date
Auscultation Method Using Brachial Artery 1. Wash hands/hand hygiene. *Comments:*	☐	☐	☐	
2. Determine which extremity is most appropriate for reading. *Comments:*	☐	☐	☐	
3. Select a cuff size appropriate for the client. *Comments:*	☐	☐	☐	
4. Rest client's bare arm on a support so the midpoint of the upper arm is at the level of the heart. Extend elbow with palm turned upward. *Comments:*	☐	☐	☐	
5. Make sure bladder cuff is fully deflated and pump valve moves freely. Place manometer at eye level and easily visible. *Comments:*	☐	☐	☐	
6. Palpate brachial artery in antecubital space, and place cuff so that midline of bladder is over arterial pulsation. Wrap and secure cuff snugly around client's bare upper arm. Lower edge of cuff should be 1 inch above antecubital fossa where head of stethoscope is to be placed. *Comments:*	☐	☐	☐	

continued on the following page

continued from the previous page

Procedure 26-4 Assessing Blood Pressure	Able to Perform	Able to Perform with Assistance	Unable to Perform	Initials/Date
7. Inflate cuff rapidly to 70 mm Hg and increase by 10-mm increments while palpating radial pulse. Note level of pressure at which pulse disappears and subsequently reappears during deflation. *Comments:*	☐	☐	☐	
8. Insert stethoscope earpieces into ear canals. *Comments:*	☐	☐	☐	
9. Relocate brachial artery with nondominant hand, and place stethoscope bell over brachial artery pulsation. *Comments:*	☐	☐	☐	
10. With dominant hand, turn valve clockwise to close. Compress pump to inflate cuff rapidly and steadily until manometer registers 20–30 mm Hg above the level previously determined by palpation. *Comments:*	☐	☐	☐	
11. Partially unscrew (open) valve counter-clockwise to deflate bladder at 2 mm/sec while listening for the 5 phases of the Korotkoff sounds. Note manometer reading for these sounds. *Comments:*	☐	☐	☐	
12. After the last Korotkoff's sound is heard, deflate cuff slowly for at least another 10 mm Hg then deflate rapidly and completely. *Comments:*	☐	☐	☐	

continued on the following page

continued from the previous page

Procedure 26-4 Assessing Blood Pressure	Able to Perform	Able to Perform with Assistance	Unable to Perform	Initials/Date
13. Allow client to rest for at least 30 seconds and remove cuff. *Comments:*	☐	☐	☐	
14. Inform client of reading. *Comments:*	☐	☐	☐	
15. Record the BP reading. *Comments:*	☐	☐	☐	
16. If appropriate, lower bed, raise side rails, and place call light in easy reach. *Comments:*	☐	☐	☐	
17. Put all equipment in proper place. *Comments:*	☐	☐	☐	
18. Wash hands/hand hygiene. *Comments:*	☐	☐	☐	

Checklist for Procedure 28-1   Performing Venipuncture (Blood Drawing)

Name _____ Date _____

School _____

Instructor _____

Course _____

Procedure 28-1 Performing Venipuncture (Blood Drawing)	Able to Perform	Able to Perform with Assistance	Unable to Perform	Initials/Date
1. Greet client by name and validate client's identification. *Comments:*	☐	☐	☐	
2. Explain the procedure to client. *Comments:*	☐	☐	☐	
3. Hand hygiene. *Comments:*	☐	☐	☐	
4. Gather equipment. *Comments:*	☐	☐	☐	
5. Close curtain or door. *Comments:*	☐	☐	☐	
6. Raise or lower bed and table to comfortable working height. *Comments:*	☐	☐	☐	
7. Position client's arm; extend arm to form a straight line from shoulder to wrist. Place pillow or towel under upper arm. Client should be in a supine or semi-Fowler's position. *Comments:*	☐	☐	☐	

continued on the following page

continued from the previous page

Procedure 28-1 **Performing Venipuncture (Blood Drawing)**	**Able to Perform**	**Able to Perform with Assistance**	**Unable to Perform**	**Initials/Date**
8. Apply disposable gloves. *Comments:*	☐	☐	☐	
9. Apply the tourniquet 3–4 inches above venipuncture site. *Comments:*	☐	☐	☐	
10. Check for the distal pulse. Reapply if no pulse detected. *Comments:*	☐	☐	☐	
11. Have client open and close fist several times, leaving fist clenched before venipuncture. *Comments:*	☐	☐	☐	
12. Maintain tourniquet for only 1–2 minutes. *Comments:*	☐	☐	☐	
13. Palpate to identify best venipuncture site. *Comments:*	☐	☐	☐	
14. Select the vein for venipuncture. *Comments:*	☐	☐	☐	
15. Prepare to obtain blood sample. Technique varies, depending on equipment used: • Syringe method: Have syringe with appropriate needle attached.	☐	☐	☐	

continued on the following page

continued from the previous page

Procedure 28-1 Performing Venipuncture (Blood Drawing)	Able to Perform	Able to Perform with Assistance	Unable to Perform	Initials/Date
• Vacutainer method: Attach double-ended needle to Vacutainer tube and have proper blood specimen tube resting inside Vacutainer. Do not puncture rubber stopper yet. *Comments:*				
16. Cleanse venipuncture site with alcohol swab or chlorhexidine alcohol, using a circular method at site and extending motion 2 inches beyond site. Allow alcohol to dry. *Comments:*	☐	☐	☐	
17. Remove needle cover and warn that client will feel needle stick for a few seconds. *Comments:*	☐	☐	☐	
18. Place thumb or forefinger of nondominant hand 1 inch below site and pull skin taut. *Comments:*	☐	☐	☐	
19. Hold syringe needle or Vacutainer at a 15° to 30° angle from skin with bevel up. *Comments:*	☐	☐	☐	
20. Slowly insert needle or Vacutainer. *Comments:*	☐	☐	☐	
21. Technique varies, depending on equipment used: • Syringe method: Gently pull back on syringe plunger and look for blood return. Obtain desired amount of blood into syringe.	☐	☐	☐	

continued on the following page

continued from the previous page

Procedure 28-1 Performing Venipuncture (Blood Drawing)	Able to Perform	Able to Perform with Assistance	Unable to Perform	Initials/Date
• Vacutainer method: Hold Vacutainer securely and advance specimen tube into holder needle. Do not advance needle into vein. After collection tube is full, grasp Vacutainer firmly, remove tube, and insert additional specimen collection tubes, as indicated. *Comments:*				
22. After specimen collection is completed, release tourniquet. *Comments:*	☐	☐	☐	
23. Apply 2 × 2 gauze over puncture site without applying pressure and quickly withdraw needle from vein. *Comments:*	☐	☐	☐	
24. Immediately apply pressure over venipuncture site with gauze for 2–3 minutes or until bleeding has stopped. Tape gauze dressing over the (or apply a Band-Aid). *Comments:*	☐	☐	☐	
25. Syringe method: Using one hand, insert syringe needle into appropriate collection tube and allow vacuum to fill. *Comments:*	☐	☐	☐	
26. If any blood tubes contain additives, gently rotate back and forth 8–10 times. *Comments:*	☐	☐	☐	

continued on the following page

continued from the previous page

Procedure 28-1 Performing Venipuncture (Blood Drawing)	Able to Perform	Able to Perform with Assistance	Unable to Perform	Initials/Date
27. Inspect client's puncture site for bleeding. Reapply clean gauze and tape, if necessary. *Comments:*	☐	☐	☐	
28. Assist client into a comfortable position. Return bed to low position with side rails up, if appropriate. *Comments:*	☐	☐	☐	
29. Check tubes for any external blood and decontaminate with alcohol, as appropriate. *Comments:*	☐	☐	☐	
30. Check tubes for proper labeling. Place tubes into appropriate bags and containers for transport to laboratory. *Comments:*	☐	☐	☐	
31. Dispose of needles, syringe, and soiled equipment into proper container. *Comments:*	☐	☐	☐	
32. Remove and dispose of gloves. *Comments:*	☐	☐	☐	
33. Wash hands/hand hygiene. *Comments:*	☐	☐	☐	
34. Send specimens to laboratory. *Comments:*	☐	☐	☐	

Checklist for Procedure 28-2 Performing a Skin Puncture

Name _____ Date _____

School _____

Instructor _____

Course _____

Procedure 28-2 Performing a Skin Puncture	Able to Perform	Able to Perform with Assistance	Unable to Perform	Initials/Date
1. Wash hands/hand hygiene. *Comments:*	☐	☐	☐	
2. Check client's identification band, if appropriate. *Comments:*	☐	☐	☐	
3. Explain procedure to client. *Comments:*	☐	☐	☐	
4. Gather equipment. *Comments:*	☐	☐	☐	
5. Apply gloves. *Comments:*	☐	☐	☐	
6. Select site. *Comments:*	☐	☐	☐	
7. Place site in a dependent position; apply warm compresses, if needed. *Comments:*	☐	☐	☐	
8. Place a hand towel or absorbent pad under extremity. *Comments:*	☐	☐	☐	

continued on the following page

continued from the previous page

Procedure 28-2 Performing a Skin Puncture	Able to Perform	Able to Perform with Assistance	Unable to Perform	Initials/Date
9. Cleanse puncture site with an antiseptic and allow to dry. *Comments:*	☐	☐	☐	
10. With nondominant hand, apply gentle milking pressure above or around puncture site. Do not touch puncture site. *Comments:*	☐	☐	☐	
11. Read directions carefully before using the lancet. • With sterile lancet at a 90° angle to skin, use a quick stab to puncture skin (about 2 mm deep). • With automatic unistik, push lancet into body of unistik until it clicks. Hold unistik body and twist off lance cap. Place end of unistik tightly against client's finger and press the lever. Needle automatically retracts after use. *Comments:*	☐	☐	☐	
12. Wipe off first drop of blood with sterile 2 × 2 gauze; allow blood to flow freely. *Comments:*	☐	☐	☐	
13. Collect blood into tube(s). If blood for a platelet count is to be collected, obtain this specimen first. *Comments:*	☐	☐	☐	
14. Apply pressure to puncture site with a sterile 2 × 2 gauze. *Comments:*	☐	☐	☐	

continued on the following page

continued from the previous page

Procedure 28-2 **Performing a Skin Puncture**	Able to Perform	Able to Perform with Assistance	Unable to Perform	Initials/Date
15. Place contaminated articles into a sharps container. *Comments:*	☐	☐	☐	
16. Remove gloves; wash hands. *Comments:*	☐	☐	☐	
17. Position client for comfort with call light in reach. *Comments:*	☐	☐	☐	
18. Wash hands/hand hygiene. *Comments:*	☐	☐	☐	

Checklist for Procedure 28-3   Obtaining a Residual Urine Specimen from an Indwelling Catheter

Name _____ Date _____

School _____

Instructor _____

Course _____

Procedure 28-3 Obtaining a Residual Urine Specimen from an Indwelling Catheter	Able to Perform	Able to Perform with Assistance	Unable to Perform	Initials/Date
1. Wash hands/hand hygiene. *Comments:*	☐	☐	☐	
2. Check prescribing practitioner's orders. *Comments:*	☐	☐	☐	
3. Explain procedure to client and provide privacy. *Comments:*	☐	☐	☐	
4. Check for urine in tubing. *Comments:*	☐	☐	☐	
5. If more urine is needed, clamp tubing using a nonserrated clamp or a rubber band for 10–15 minutes. *Comments:*	☐	☐	☐	
6. Put on clean gloves. *Comments:*	☐	☐	☐	
7. Clean sample port with a povidone-iodine swab. *Comments:*	☐	☐	☐	

continued on the following page

continued from the previous page

Procedure 28-3 **Obtaining a Residual Urine Specimen from an Indwelling Catheter**	**Able to Perform**	**Able to Perform with Assistance**	**Unable to Perform**	**Initials/Date**
8. Insert sterile needle and syringe into sample port or catheter at a 45° angle and withdraw 10 ml of urine. *Comments:*	☐	☐	☐	
9. Put urine into sterile container and close tightly, taking care not to contaminate container lid. *Comments:*	☐	☐	☐	
10. Remove clamp and rearrange tubing, avoiding dependent loops. *Comments:*	☐	☐	☐	
11. Label specimen container, put in a plastic bag, and send to laboratory. *Comments:*	☐	☐	☐	
12. Wash hands/hand hygiene. *Comments:*	☐	☐	☐	

Checklist for Procedure 28-4   Collecting a Clean-Catch, Midstream Urine Specimen

Name _____ Date _____

School _____

Instructor _____

Course _____

Procedure 28-4 Collecting a Clean-Catch, Midstream Urine Specimen	Able to Perform	Able to Perform with Assistance	Unable to Perform	Initials/Date
1. Check orders and assess need for the procedure. *Comments:*	☐	☐	☐	
2. Gather equipment. Wash hands/hand hygiene. *Comments:*	☐	☐	☐	
3. Assess client's ability to complete procedure, including understanding, mobility, and balance. *Comments:*	☐	☐	☐	
4. Assess client for signs and symptoms of urinary abnormalities. *Comments:*	☐	☐	☐	
5. Check client's identification. *Comments:*	☐	☐	☐	
6. If client is to complete procedure in privacy, explain procedure, give equipment to client, and wait for specimen. If client has decreased personal hygiene, perform procedure after a bath or have client wash the perineal area before a procedure. *Comments:*	☐	☐	☐	

continued on the following page

continued from the previous page

Procedure 28-4 Collecting a Clean-Catch, Midstream Urine Specimen	Able to Perform	Able to Perform with Assistance	Unable to Perform	Initials/Date
7. If nurse is to perform procedure: Wash hands and apply gloves. If client is to perform procedure, instruct client to wash hands before and after procedure. If more comfortable, allow client to wear gloves. *Comments:*	☐	☐	☐	
8. Provide privacy. *Comments:*	☐	☐	☐	
9. Instruct client on positioning. *Comments:*	☐	☐	☐	
10. Using sterile procedure, open kit or towelettes. Open sterile container, placing lid with sterile side up on a firm surface. *Comments:*	☐	☐	☐	
11. Female client: • Use thumb and forefinger to separate labia, or have client separate labia with fingers. • Use a downward stroke and cleanse one side of labia with towelette. Discard towelette. • Repeat on other side. • With a third towelette, use a downward stroke from the top to bottom of urethral opening. Discard towelette. *Comments:*	☐	☐	☐	

continued on the following page

continued from the previous page

Procedure 28-4 **Collecting a Clean-Catch, Midstream Urine Specimen**	**Able to Perform**	**Able to Perform with Assistance**	**Unable to Perform**	**Initials/Date**
12. Male client: • Pull back foreskin (if present) and clean with a single stroke around meatus and glans. • Use a circular motion, starting with head of penis at urethral opening, moving down glans shaft. Discard towelette. • Cleanse head of penis three times using a circular motion. Use a new towelette each time. *Comments:*	☐	☐	☐	
13. Ask client to begin to urinate into the toilet. After stream starts with good flow, place collection cup under urine stream. Avoid touching skin with container. Fill container with 30–60 cc of urine and remove container before urination ceases. *Comments:*	☐	☐	☐	
14. Place sterile lid back onto container and close tightly. Clean and dry outside of container with a towelette. Wash hands. Label and enclose in a plastic biohazard bag and follow facility policy for transporting specimen to laboratory. *Comments:*	☐	☐	☐	
15. Remove and dispose of gloves; wash hands/hand hygiene. *Comments:*	☐	☐	☐	

Checklist for Procedure 28-5   Measuring Blood Glucose Levels

Name _____ Date _____

School _____

Instructor _____

Course _____

Procedure 28-5 Measuring Blood Glucose Levels	Able to Perform	Able to Perform with Assistance	Unable to Perform	Initials/Date
1. Review orders, identify client, and review manufacturer's instructions for meter usage. *Comments:*	☐	☐	☐	
2. Wash hands/hand hygiene. *Comments:*	☐	☐	☐	
3. Assemble equipment at bedside. *Comments:*	☐	☐	☐	
4. Have client wash hands wth soap and water and position client comfortably in a semi-Fowler's position or upright in a chair. *Comments:*	☐	☐	☐	
5. Remove a reagent strip from container and reseal container cap. Turn on meter. *Comments:*	☐	☐	☐	
6. Following manufacturer's instructions, calibrate meter, if needed. *Comments:*	☐	☐	☐	
7. Remove unused reagent strip from meter and place on a clean, dry surface (paper towel) with test pad facing up. *Comments:*	☐	☐	☐	

continued on the following page

continued from the previous page

Procedure 28-5 **Measuring Blood Glucose Levels**	**Able to Perform**	**Able to Perform with Assistance**	**Unable to Perform**	**Initials/Date**
8. Apply disposable gloves. *Comments:*	☐	☐	☐	
9. Select appropriate puncture site and perform skin puncture. *Comments:*	☐	☐	☐	
10. Wipe away first drop of blood from site. *Comments:*	☐	☐	☐	
11. Gently squeeze site to produce a droplet of blood. *Comments:*	☐	☐	☐	
12. Transfer drop of blood to reagent strip by carefully moving site over strip. *Comments:*	☐	☐	☐	
13. Quickly press meter timer according to manufacturer's instructions. *Comments:*	☐	☐	☐	
14. Apply pressure to puncture site. *Comments:*	☐	☐	☐	
15. According to manufacturer's instructions, wipe blood from test pad with a cotton ball; place strip into meter. Allow timer to continue. *Comments:*	☐	☐	☐	

continued on the following page

continued from the previous page

Procedure 28-5 **Measuring Blood Glucose Levels**	**Able to Perform**	**Able to Perform with Assistance**	**Unable to Perform**	**Initials/Date**
16. Read meter for results found on the unit display. *Comments:*	☐	☐	☐	
17. Turn off meter and properly dispose of the test strip, cotton ball, and lancet. *Comments:*	☐	☐	☐	
18. Remove disposable gloves and place them in appropriate receptacle. *Comments:*	☐	☐	☐	
19. Wash hands/hand hygiene. *Comments:*	☐	☐	☐	
20. Review test results with client. *Comments:*	☐	☐	☐	
21. Notify prescribing practitioner of test results. *Comments:*	☐	☐	☐	
22. Wash hands/hand hygiene. *Comments:*	☐	☐	☐	

Checklist for Procedure 29-1   Applying Restraints

Name _____ Date _____

School _____

Instructor _____

Course _____

Procedure 29-1 Applying Restraints	Able to Perform	Able to Perform with Assistance	Unable to Perform	Initials/Date
Chest Restraint 1. Wash hands/hand hygiene. *Comments:*	☐	☐	☐	
2. Explain that client will be wearing a jacket attached to the bed for safety. Follow institutional policy regarding restraint use. *Comments:*	☐	☐	☐	
3. Place restraint over client's hospital gown or clothing. *Comments:*	☐	☐	☐	
4. Place restraint on client with opening in front. *Comments:*	☐	☐	☐	
5. Overlap front pieces, threading ties through slot or loop on vest front. *Comments:*	☐	☐	☐	
6. If client is in bed, secure ties to movable part of mattress frame with a half-knot. *Comments:*	☐	☐	☐	

continued on the following page

continued from the previous page

Procedure 29-1 Applying Restraints	Able to Perform	Able to Perform with Assistance	Unable to Perform	Initials/Date
7. If client is in a chair, cross straps behind seat of chair and secure straps to chair's lower legs, out of client's reach. If in a wheelchair, be sure straps will not get caught up in wheels. *Comments:*	☐	☐	☐	
8. Step back and assess client's overall safety. Be sure restraint is loose enough not to be a hazard to client but tight enough to restrict client from getting up and harming self. *Comments:*	☐	☐	☐	
9. Wash hands/hand hygiene. *Comments:*	☐	☐	☐	
Applying Wrist or Ankle Restraints 1. Wash hands/hand hygiene. *Comments:*	☐	☐	☐	
2. Explain to client that you will be placing a wrist or ankle band that will restrict movement. Follow institutional policy regarding restraint use. *Comments:*	☐	☐	☐	
3. Place padding around client's wrist or ankle. *Comments:*	☐	☐	☐	
4. Wrap restraint around client's wrist or ankle, pulling tie through loop in restraint and tying a square knot. *Comments:*	☐	☐	☐	

continued on the following page

continued from the previous page

Procedure 29-1 Applying Restraints	Able to Perform	Able to Perform with Assistance	Unable to Perform	Initials/Date
5. Tie restraint ties to movable portion of mattress frame. *Comments:*	☐	☐	☐	.
6. Slip two fingers under restraint to check for tightness. Be sure restraint is tight enough that client cannot slip it off but loose enough that neurovascular status of client's extremity is not impaired. *Comments:*	☐	☐	☐	
7. Step back and assess client's overall safety. Be sure restraint is loose enough not to be a hazard to client but tight enough to restrict client from getting up and harming self. *Comments:*	☐	☐	☐	
8. Place call light within client's reach. *Comments:*	☐	☐	☐	
9. Check on client every half hour while restrained. Assess safety of restraint placement and client's neurovascular status. *Comments:*	☐	☐	☐	
10. Wash hands/hand hygiene. *Comments:*	☐	☐	☐	

Checklist for Procedure 29-2   Handwashing: Visibly Soiled Hands

Name _____ Date _____

School _____

Instructor _____

Course _____

Procedure 29-2 **Handwashing: Visibly Soiled Hands**	Able to Perform	Able to Perform with Assistance	Unable to Perform	Initials/Date
1. Remove jewelry. Wristwatch can be pushed up above wrist (midforearm). Push sleeves of uniform or shirt up above wrist at midforearm level. *Comments:*	☐	☐	☐	
2. Assess hands for hangnails, cuts or breaks in skin, and areas that are heavily soiled. *Comments:*	☐	☐	☐	
3. Turn on water. Adjust flow and temperature. Water temperature should be warm. *Comments:*	☐	☐	☐	
4. Wet hands and lower forearms thoroughly by holding under running water. Keep hands and forearms in down position with elbows straight. Avoid splashing water and touching sides of sink. *Comments:*	☐	☐	☐	
5. Apply about 5 ml (1 teaspoon) of liquid soap. Lather thoroughly. *Comments:*	☐	☐	☐	
6. Vigorously rub hands together for 15 seconds. *Comments:*	☐	☐	☐	

continued on the following page

continued from the previous page

Procedure 29-2 Handwashing: Visibly Soiled Hands	Able to Perform	Able to Perform with Assistance	Unable to Perform	Initials/Date
7. Rinse with hands in down position, elbows straight, in direction of forearm to wrist to fingers. *Comments:*	☐	☐	☐	
8. Blot hands and forearms to dry thoroughly. Dry in direction of fingers to wrist and forearms. Discard paper towels in proper receptacle. *Comments:*	☐	☐	☐	
9. Turn off water faucet with a clean, dry paper towel. *Comments:*	☐	☐	☐	

Checklist for Procedure 29-3   Applying Sterile Gloves via the Open Method

Name _____ Date _____

School _____

Instructor _____

Course _____

Procedure 29-3 Applying Sterile Gloves via the Open Method	Able to Perform	Able to Perform with Assistance	Unable to Perform	Initials/Date
1. Wash hands/hand hygiene. *Comments:*	☐	☐	☐	
2. Place inner wrapper onto a clean, dry surface. Open inner wrapper to expose gloves. *Comments:*	☐	☐	☐	
3. Identify right and left hand; glove dominant hand first. *Comments:*	☐	☐	☐	
4. Grasp cuff with thumb and first two fingers of nondominant hand, touching only inside of cuff. *Comments:*	☐	☐	☐	
5. Pull glove over dominant hand, making sure thumb and fingers fit into proper spaces. *Comments:*	☐	☐	☐	
6. With the gloved dominant hand, slip fingers under cuff of other glove, gloved thumb abducted, making sure it does not touch any part on nondominant hand. *Comments:*	☐	☐	☐	

continued on the following page

continued from the previous page

Procedure 29-3 Applying Sterile Gloves via the Open Method	Able to Perform	Able to Perform with Assistance	Unable to Perform	Initials/Date
7. Slip the glove onto nondominant hand, making sure fingers slip into proper spaces. *Comments:*	☐	☐	☐	
8. With gloved hands, interlock fingers to fit gloves onto each finger. • If gloves are soiled, remove by turning inside out as described in the following Actions: *Comments:*	☐	☐	☐	
9. Slip gloved fingers of dominant hand under cuff of opposite hand or grasp outer part of glove at wrist if there is no cuff. *Comments:*	☐	☐	☐	
10. Pull glove down to fingers, exposing thumb. *Comments:*	☐	☐	☐	
11. Slip uncovered thumb into opposite glove at wrist, allowing only glove-covered fingers of hand to touch soiled glove. *Comments:*	☐	☐	☐	
12. Pull glove down over dominant hand almost to fingertips and slip glove on to other hand. *Comments:*	☐	☐	☐	

continued on the following page

continued from the previous page

Procedure 29-3 Applying Sterile Gloves via the Open Method	Able to Perform	Able to Perform with Assistance	Unable to Perform	Initials/Date
13. With dominant hand touching only inside of other glove, pull glove over dominant hand so that only the inside (clean surface) is exposed. *Comments:*	☐	☐	☐	
14. Dispose of soiled gloves. *Comments:*	☐	☐	☐	
15. Wash hands/hand hygiene. *Comments:*	☐	☐	☐	

Checklist for Procedure 29-4 Donning and Removing Clean and Contaminated Gloves, Cap, and Mask

Name _____ Date _____

School _____

Instructor _____

Course _____

Procedure 29-4 Donning and Removing Clean and Contaminated Gloves, Cap, and Mask	Able to Perform	Able to Perform with Assistance	Unable to Perform	Initials/Date
1. Wash hands/hand hygiene. Comments:	☐	☐	☐	
2. Don cap or surgical hat or hood first. Hair should be tucked and covered so that all hair is covered. Comments:	☐	☐	☐	
3. Apply a mask around mouth and nose and secure to prevent venting. Comments:	☐	☐	☐	
4. Open gown, slip arms into sleeves, and secure at neck and side. Comments:	☐	☐	☐	
5. Wear protective eyewear, goggles or glasses, or face shields. Comments:	☐	☐	☐	
6. Apply clean gloves. If sterile gloves are required for a procedure, use open or closed method. Comments:	☐	☐	☐	
7. Open glove technique: a. Slide hands into gown through cuffs on gown. b. Pick up cuff of left glove using thumb and index finger of right hand.	☐	☐	☐	

continued on the following page

continued from the previous page

Procedure 29-4 Donning and Removing Clean and Contaminated Gloves, Cap, and Mask	Able to Perform	Able to Perform with Assistance	Unable to Perform	Initials/Date
c. Pull glove onto left hand, leaving cuff of glove turned down. d. Take gloved left hand and slide fingers inside cuff of right glove, keeping gloved fingers under folded cuff. e. Pull glove onto right hand. f. Rotate arm as cuff of glove is pulled over gown. *Comments:*				
8. Closed glove technique: a. Slide hands into gown through cuffs on gown. b. Use right hand to pick up left glove. c. Place glove on upward-turned left hand—palm side down, thumb to thumb with fingers extending along forearm pointing toward elbow. d. Hold glove cuff and sleeve cuff together with thumb of left hand. e. Right hand stretches cuff of left glove over opened end of sleeve. f. Work fingers into glove as cuff is pulled onto wrist. g. Left glove is donned in same manner. *Comments:*	☐	☐	☐	
9. Enter client's room and explain rationale for wearing isolation attire. *Comments:*	☐	☐	☐	
10. After performing necessary tasks, remove gown, gloves, mask, and cap before leaving room. *Comments:*	☐	☐	☐	

continued on the following page

continued from the previous page

Procedure 29-4 **Donning and Removing Clean and Contaminated Gloves, Cap, and Mask**	Able to Perform	Able to Perform with Assistance	Unable to Perform	Initials/Date
11. Removal of gown: Untie gown and remove from shoulders. Fold and roll gown down in front into a ball, so contaminated area is rolled onto center of gown. Dispose in approved receptacle. *Comments:*	☐	☐	☐	
12. Removal of gloves: a. Grasp outside cuff of one glove and pull off, turning inside out. Hold with remaining gloved hand. b. Pull second glove off without touching outside of second glove. Turn second glove as it is removed. Dispose into receptacle with first glove. *Comments:*	☐	☐	☐	
13. Removal of mask: Untie bottom strings of mask first, then top strings, and lift off face. Hold mask by strings and discard. *Comments:*	☐	☐	☐	
14. Removal of cap: grasp top surface of cap and lift from head. *Comments:*	☐	☐	☐	
15. Wash hands/hand hygiene. *Comments:*	☐	☐	☐	

Checklist for Procedure 29-5   Surgical Hand Antisepsis

Name _____ Date _____

School _____

Instructor _____

Course _____

Procedure 29-5 Surgical Hand Antisepsis	Able to Perform	Able to Perform with Assistance	Unable to Perform	Initials/Date
1. Remove rings, watches, and bracelets before beginning surgical scrub. *Comments:*	☐	☐	☐	
2. Use a deep sink with side or foot pedal to dispense antimicrobial soap and control water temperature and flow. *Comments:*	☐	☐	☐	
3. Have two surgical scrub brushes and nail file. *Comments:*	☐	☐	☐	
4. Apply surgical shoe covers and a cap to cover hair and ears completely. *Comments:*	☐	☐	☐	
5. Apply mask. *Comments:*	☐	☐	☐	
6. Before beginning surgical scrub: a. Open sterile package containing gown; using aseptic technique, make a sterile field with inside of gown's wrapper. b. Open sterile towel and drop it onto center of field.	☐	☐	☐	

continued on the following page

continued from the previous page

Procedure 29-5 Surgical Hand Antisepsis	Able to Perform	Able to Perform with Assistance	Unable to Perform	Initials/Date
c. Open outer wrapper from sterile gloves and drop inner package of gloves onto sterile field beside folded gown and towel. *Comments:*				
7. At a deep sink under warm, flowing water, wet hands, beginning at tips of fingers, to forearms—keeping hands at level above elbows. Prewash hands and forearms to 2 inches above elbow. *Comments:*	☐	☐	☐	
8. Apply liberal amount of soap onto hands and rub hands and arms to 2 inches above elbows. *Comments:*	☐	☐	☐	
9. Use nail file under running water; clean under each nail of both hands, and drop file into sink when finished. *Comments:*	☐	☐	☐	
10. Wet and apply soap to scrub brush, if needed. Open prepackaged scrub brush, if available. Hold brush in dominant hand, use a circular motion to scrub nails and all skin areas of nondominant hand and arm (10 strokes to each of following areas): a. Nails b. Palm of hand and anterior side of fingers. *Comments:*	☐	☐	☐	

continued on the following page

continued from the previous page

Procedure 29-5 Surgical Hand Antisepsis	Able to Perform	Able to Perform with Assistance	Unable to Perform	Initials/Date
11. Rinse brush thoroughly and reapply soap. *Comments:*	☐	☐	☐	
12. Continue to scrub nondominant arm with a circular motion for 10 strokes each to lower, middle, and upper arm; drop brush into sink. *Comments:*	☐	☐	☐	
13. Maintaining hands and arms above elbow level, place fingertips under running water and thoroughly rinse fingers, hands, and arms (allow water to run off elbow into sink); take care not to get uniform wet. *Comments:*	☐	☐	☐	
14. Take second scrub brush and repeat Actions 10–13 on dominant hand and arm. *Comments:*	☐	☐	☐	
15. Keep arms flexed and proceed to area (operating or procedure room) with sterile items. *Comments:*	☐	☐	☐	
16. Secure sterile towel by grasping it on one edge, opening towel, full length, making sure it does not touch uniform. *Comments:*	☐	☐	☐	

continued on the following page

continued from the previous page

Procedure 29-5 Surgical Hand Antisepsis	Able to Perform	Able to Perform with Assistance	Unable to Perform	Initials/Date
17. Dry each hand and arm separately; extend one side of towel around fingers and hand and dry in a rotating motion up to elbow. *Comments:*	☐	☐	☐	
18. Reverse towel and repeat same action on other hand and arm, thoroughly drying skin. *Comments:*	☐	☐	☐	
19. Discard towel into a linen hamper. *Comments:*	☐	☐	☐	

Checklist for Procedure 29-6   Applying Sterile Gloves and Gown via the Closed Method

Name _____ Date _____

School _____

Instructor _____

Course _____

Procedure 29-6 Applying Sterile Gloves and Gown via the Closed Method	Able to Perform	Able to Perform with Assistance	Unable to Perform	Initials/Date
Gowning 1. Wash hands/hand hygiene. *Comments:*	☐	☐	☐	
2. Sterile gown is folded inside out. *Comments:*	☐	☐	☐	
3. Grasp gown inside neckline, step back, and allow gown to open in front of you; keep inside of gown toward you; do not allow it to touch anything. *Comments:*	☐	☐	☐	
4. With hands at shoulder level, slip both arms into gown; keep hands inside sleeves of gown. *Comments:*	☐	☐	☐	
5. Circulating nurse will step up behind you and grasp inside of gown, bring it over your shoulders, and secure ties at neck and waist. *Comments:*	☐	☐	☐	
Closed Gloving 6. With hands still inside gown sleeves, open inner wrapper of gloves on sterile gown field. *Comments:*	☐	☐	☐	

continued on the following page

continued from the previous page

Procedure 29-6 Applying Sterile Gloves and Gown via the Closed Method	Able to Perform	Able to Perform with Assistance	Unable to Perform	Initials/Date
7. With nondominant sleeved hand, grasp glove cuff for dominant hand and lay it on extended dominant forearm; with palm up; place palm of glove against sleeved palm, with fingers of glove pointing toward elbow. *Comments:*	☐	☐	☐	
8. Manipulate glove so that sleeved thumb of dominant hand is grasping cuff; with nondominant hand, turn cuff over end of dominant hand and gown's cuff. *Comments:*	☐	☐	☐	
9. With sleeved nondominant hand, grasp glove cuff and gown's sleeve of dominant hand; slowly extend fingers into glove, making sure glove cuff remains above gown sleeve cuff. *Comments:*	☐	☐	☐	
10. With gloved dominant hand, repeat Actions 7 and 8. *Comments:*	☐	☐	☐	
11. Interlock gloved fingers; secure fit. *Comments:*	☐	☐	☐	
12. Wash hands/hand hygiene. *Comments:*	☐	☐	☐	

Checklist for Procedure 29-7   Removing Contaminated Items

Name _____ Date _____

School _____

Instructor _____

Course _____

Procedure 29-7 Removing Contaminated Items	Able to Perform	Able to Perform with Assistance	Unable to Perform	Initials/Date
Removal of Soiled Linen 1. Wash hands/hand hygiene. *Comments:*	☐	☐	☐	
2. Wear disposable gloves; wear other protective items (gowns, goggles), as determined by situation and insititution's policies. *Comments:*	☐	☐	☐	
3. Place labeled linen bag in stand. *Comments:*	☐	☐	☐	
4. Gather linens and separate from disposable items. *Comments:*	☐	☐	☐	
5. Do not allow linens to touch floor. *Comments:*	☐	☐	☐	
6. Place soiled linens in linen bag; keep clean linens in a different area. *Comments:*	☐	☐	☐	
7. Take care not to shake linens when removing items from bed or bathroom. *Comments:*	☐	☐	☐	

continued on the following page

continued from the previous page

Procedure 29-7 Removing Contaminated Items	Able to Perform	Able to Perform with Assistance	Unable to Perform	Initials/Date
8. Do not allow soiled linens to come into contact with clothing. Carry linens with arms extended outward. *Comments:*	☐	☐	☐	
9. Do not overfill linen bag. *Comments:*	☐	☐	☐	
10. Tie ends of linen bag securely. *Comments:*	☐	☐	☐	
11. Check for any punctures or tears in linen bag. *Comments:*	☐	☐	☐	
12. Double bag items if concerned that outside of bag is contaminated or torn. *Comments:*	☐	☐	☐	
13. Wash hands/hand hygiene. *Comments:*	☐	☐	☐	
Double-Bagging Technique 14. Follow Actions 1–11. Place first bag into second bag. *Comments:*	☐	☐	☐	
15. Label and secure second bag. *Comments:*	☐	☐	☐	
16. Linens are then ready for laundry. *Comments:*	☐	☐	☐	

continued on the following page

continued from the previous page

Procedure 29-7 Removing Contaminated Items	Able to Perform	Able to Perform with Assistance	Unable to Perform	Initials/Date
17. Wash hands/hand hygiene. *Comments:*	☐	☐	☐	
Removal of Other Contaminated Items 18. Follow same procedure as for all linens when removing and bagging trash. *Comments:*	☐	☐	☐	
19. Change sharps container when three quarters full or if outside of container becomes contaminated. Lock down lid of sharps container, if available, and follow hospital policy for removal. Never reach into a container. *Comments:*	☐	☐	☐	
20. Wash hands/hand hygiene. *Comments:*	☐	☐	☐	
21. Use disposable equipment when able. *Comments:*	☐	☐	☐	
22. Properly bag, label, and remove any nondisposable equipment that requires special cleaning (disinfection and sterilization). *Comments:*	☐	☐	☐	
23. Disassemble special procedure trays into disposable and nondisposable parts. Send nondisposable items (after proper bagging) to central services for decontamination. *Comments:*	☐	☐	☐	

continued on the following page

continued from the previous page

Procedure 29-7 Removing Contaminated Items	Able to Perform	Able to Perform with Assistance	Unable to Perform	Initials/Date
24. Place laboratory specimens in a leak-proof container. Check to see that containers are not visibly contaminated on outside. *Comments:*	☐	☐	☐	
25. Wash hands/hand hygiene. *Comments:*	☐	☐	☐	

Checklist for Procedure 29-8 Bathing a Client in Bed

Name _____ Date _____

School _____

Instructor _____

Course _____

Procedure 29-8 Bathing a Client in Bed	Able to Perform	Able to Perform with Assistance	Unable to Perform	Initials/Date
1. Assess client's preferences about bathing. *Comments:*	☐	☐	☐	
2. Explain procedure to client. Gather supplies. *Comments:*	☐	☐	☐	
3. Prepare environment. Close doors and windows, adjust temperature, provide time for elimination needs and for privacy. *Comments:*	☐	☐	☐	
4. Wash hands/hand hygiene. Apply gloves. Change gloves when emptying water basin. *Comments:*	☐	☐	☐	
5. Lower side rail on side close to you. Position client in a comfortable position closest to side near you. *Comments:*	☐	☐	☐	
6. If available, place bath blanket over top sheet. Remove top sheet from under bath blanket. Remove client's gown. Fold bath blanket to expose only area being cleaned at that time. *Comments:*	☐	☐	☐	

continued on the following page

continued from the previous page

Procedure 29-8 Bathing a Client in Bed	Able to Perform	Able to Perform with Assistance	Unable to Perform	Initials/Date
7. Fill washbasin two thirds full. Permit client to test temperature of water with hand. Change water when a soap film develops or water becomes soiled. *Comments:*	☐	☐	☐	
8. Wet washcloth and wring it out. *Comments:*	☐	☐	☐	
9. Make bath mitten with washcloth. *Comments:*	☐	☐	☐	
10. Wash client's face. Use a separate corner of washcloth for each eye, wiping from inner to outer canthus. Wash neck and ears. Rinse and pat dry. Male clients may want to shave at this time. Provide assistance with shaving as needed. *Comments:*	☐	☐	☐	
11. Wash arms, forearms, and hands, using long, firm strokes distal to proximal. Wash axilla. Rinse and pat dry. Apply deodorant or powder if client desires. Allow hand to soak about 3–5 minutes, then wash hands, interdigit area, fingers, and fingernails. Rinse and pat dry. *Comments:*	☐	☐	☐	
12. Wash chest and abdomen. Fold bath blanket down to umbilicus. Wash chest using long, firm strokes. Wash skin fold under female client's breast by lifting each breast. Rinse and pat dry. Wash abdomen using long, firm strokes. Rinse and pat dry. Cover chest or abdomen area in between washing, rinsing, and drying to prevent chilling. *Comments:*	☐	☐	☐	

continued on the following page

continued from the previous page

Procedure 29-8 Bathing a Client in Bed	Able to Perform	Able to Perform with Assistance	Unable to Perform	Initials/Date
13. Wash legs and feet. Expose leg farthest from you by folding bath blanket to midline. Place washbasin on bath towel in bed. Place client's foot into washbasin. Allow foot to soak while washing leg with long, firm strokes in direction of distal to proximal. Rinse and pat dry. Clean soles, interdigits, and toes. Rinse and pat dry. Perform same with other leg and foot. *Comments:*	☐	☐	☐	
14. Wash back. Rinse and pat dry. Give back rub and apply lotion. *Comments:*	☐	☐	☐	
15. Perineal care: Assist client to supine position. Perform perineal care. *Comments:*	☐	☐	☐	
16. Apply lotion as desired or needed. Apply clean gown. *Comments:*	☐	☐	☐	
17. Document skin assessment, type of bath given, and client outcomes and responses. *Comments:*	☐	☐	☐	
18. Wash hands/hand hygiene. *Comments:*	☐	☐	☐	

Checklist for Procedure 29-9   Changing Linens in an Unoccupied Bed

Name _____ Date _____

School _____

Instructor _____

Course _____

Procedure 29-9 Changing Linens in an Unoccupied Bed	Able to Perform	Able to Perform with Assistance	Unable to Perform	Initials/Date
1. Wash hands/hand hygiene. *Comments:*	☐	☐	☐	
2. Place hamper by client's door if linen bags are needed. Assess condition of blanket and bedspread. Explain procedure to client. *Comments:*	☐	☐	☐	
3. Gather linens and gloves. Place linens on clean, dry surface in reverse order of usage. *Comments:*	☐	☐	☐	
4. Apply gloves. *Comments:*	☐	☐	☐	
5. Inquire about client's toileting needs and attend as necessary. *Comments:*	☐	☐	☐	
6. Assist client to safe, comfortable chair. *Comments:*	☐	☐	☐	
7. Position bed flat: side rails down, adjust height to waist level. *Comments:*	☐	☐	☐	

continued on the following page

continued from the previous page

Procedure 29-9 Changing Linens in an Unoccupied Bed	Able to Perform	Able to Perform with Assistance	Unable to Perform	Initials/Date
8. Remove and fold blanket or bedspread. If clean and reusable, place on clean work area. *Comments:*	☐	☐	☐	
9. Remove soiled pillowcases by grasping closed end with one hand and slipping pillow out with the other. Place pillows on clean work area. *Comments:*	☐	☐	☐	
10. Remove soiled linens. *Comments:*	☐	☐	☐	
11. Fold soiled linens. Place in linen bag, keeping soiled linens away from uniform. *Comments:*	☐	☐	☐	
12. Check mattress. If soiled, clean with an antiseptic solution and dry thoroughly. *Comments:*	☐	☐	☐	
13. Remove gloves, wash hands, and apply second pair of clean gloves (when appropriate). *Comments:*	☐	☐	☐	
14. Apply clean mattress pad. *Comments:*	☐	☐	☐	
15. Place bottom sheet onto mattress. *Comments:*	☐	☐	☐	

continued on the following page

continued from the previous page

Procedure 29-9 Changing Linens in an Unoccupied Bed	Able to Perform	Able to Perform with Assistance	Unable to Perform	Initials/Date
Fitted Bottom Sheet 16. Position self diagonally toward head of bed. *Comments:*	☐	☐	☐	
17. Start at head with seamed side of fitted sheet toward mattress. *Comments:*	☐	☐	☐	
18. Lift mattress corner closest to bed; with other hand, pull and tuck fitted sheet over mattress corner; secure at head of bed. *Comments:*	☐	☐	☐	
19. Pull and tuck fitted sheet over mattress corners at foot of bed. *Comments:*	☐	☐	☐	
Flat Regular Sheet 20. Unfold bottom sheet with seamed side toward mattress. Align bottom edge of sheet with edge of mattress at foot of bed. *Comments:*	☐	☐	☐	
21. Allow sheet to hang 10 inches over mattress on side and at top. *Comments:*	☐	☐	☐	
22. Position self diagonally toward head of bed. Tuck sheet under mattress. *Comments:*	☐	☐	☐	
23. Miter sheet corner at head of bed using Actions 24–26. *Comments:*	☐	☐	☐	

continued on the following page

continued from the previous page

Procedure 29-9 Changing Linens in an Unoccupied Bed	Able to Perform	Able to Perform with Assistance	Unable to Perform	Initials/Date
24. Face side of bed and lift and lay top edge of sheet onto bed to form a triangular fold. *Comments:*	☐	☐	☐	
25. With palms down, tuck lower edge of sheet under mattress. *Comments:*	☐	☐	☐	
26. Grasp triangular fold, bring it down over side of mattress. Allow sheet to hang free at side of mattress. *Comments:*	☐	☐	☐	
27. Place draw sheet on bottom sheet and unfold it to middle crease. *Comments:*	☐	☐	☐	
28. Face side of bed, palms of hands down. Tuck both bottom and draw sheets under mattress. *Comments:*	☐	☐	☐	
29. Repeat actions on other side of bed. *Comments:*	☐	☐	☐	
30. Unfold draw sheet, if used, and grasp free-hanging sides of both bottom and draw sheets. Pull toward you, keeping back straight, and with a firm grasp, tuck both sheets under mattress. Place protective pad on bottom sheet. *Comments:*	☐	☐	☐	

continued on the following page

continued from the previous page

Procedure 29-9 Changing Linens in an Unoccupied Bed	Able to Perform	Able to Perform with Assistance	Unable to Perform	Initials/Date
31. Place top sheet on bed and unfold lengthwise, placing center crease (width) of sheet in middle of bed. Place top edge of sheet (seam up) even with top of mattress at head of bed. Pull remaining length toward bottom of bed. *Comments:*	☐	☐	☐	
32. Unfold and apply blanket or spread. Follow same technique as used in applying top sheet. *Comments:*	☐	☐	☐	
33. Miter bottom corners, as described above. Tuck lower edge of sheet under mattress. *Comments:*	☐	☐	☐	
34. Face head of bed and fold top sheet and blanket over 6 inches. Fanfold sheet and blanket (from foot to middle of bed). *Comments:*	☐	☐	☐	
35. Apply clean pillowcase on each pillow. *Comments:*	☐	☐	☐	
36. Return bed to lowest position and elevate head of bed 30° to 45°. Put side rails up on side farthest from client. *Comments:*	☐	☐	☐	
37. Inquire about toileting needs of client; assist as necessary. *Comments:*	☐	☐	☐	

continued on the following page

continued from the previous page

Procedure 29-9 Changing Linens in an Unoccupied Bed	Able to Perform	Able to Perform with Assistance	Unable to Perform	Initials/Date
38. Assist client back into bed and pull up side rails; place call light in reach; take vital signs. *Comments:*	☐	☐	☐	
39. Remove gloves; wash hand/hand hygiene. *Comments:*	☐	☐	☐	
40. Document your actions and client's response during procedure and to sitting up in chair. *Comments:*	☐	☐	☐	

Checklist for Procedure 29-10 Changing Linens in an Occupied Bed

Name _____ Date _____

School _____

Instructor _____

Course _____

Procedure 29-10 Changing Linens in an Occupied Bed	Able to Perform	Able to Perform with Assistance	Unable to Perform	Initials/Date
1. Explain procedure to client and gather equipment. *Comments:*	☐	☐	☐	
2. Wash hands/hand hygiene. *Comments:*	☐	☐	☐	
3. Bring equipment to bedside. *Comments:*	☐	☐	☐	
4. Remove top sheet and blanket. Cover client with bath blanket, if necessary. *Comments:*	☐	☐	☐	
5. Position client on side, facing away from you. Reposition pillow under head. *Comments:*	☐	☐	☐	
6. Fanfold or roll bottom linens close to client toward center of bed. *Comments:*	☐	☐	☐	
7. Smooth wrinkles out of mattress. Place clean bottom linens with center fold nearest client. Fanfold or roll clean bottom linens nearest client and tuck under soiled linens. *Comments:*	☐	☐	☐	

continued on the following page

continued from the previous page

Procedure 29-10 Changing Linens in an Occupied Bed	Able to Perform	Able to Perform with Assistance	Unable to Perform	Initials/Date
8. Miter bottom sheet. Tuck sides of sheet under mattress. *Comments:*	☐	☐	☐	
9. Fold draw sheet in half. Place center of draw sheet close to client. Fanfold or roll draw sheet closest to client and tuck under soiled linens. Smooth linens. Add protective padding, if needed. Tuck draw sheet under mattress, working from center to edges. *Comments:*	☐	☐	☐	
10. Logroll client over onto side facing you. Raise side rail. *Comments:*	☐	☐	☐	
11. Move to other side of bed. Remove soiled linens by rolling into a bundle and place in linen hamper without touching uniform. *Comments:*	☐	☐	☐	
12. Unfold or unroll bottom sheet, then draw sheet. Look for objects left in bed. Grasp each sheet with knuckles up and over sheet and pull tightly while leaning back with body weight. Client can be positioned supine. *Comments:*	☐	☐	☐	
13. Place top sheet over client with center of sheet in middle of bed. Unfold top of sheet over client. Remove bath blankets left on client to prevent exposure during bed making. Place top blanket over client, same as top sheet. *Comments:*	☐	☐	☐	

continued on the following page

continued from the previous page

Procedure 29-10 **Changing Linens in an Occupied Bed**	**Able to Perform**	**Able to Perform with Assistance**	**Unable to Perform**	**Initials/Date**
14. Raise foot of mattress and tuck top sheet and blanket under. Miter the corner. *Comments:*	☐	☐	☐	
15. Grasp top sheet and blanket over client's toes and pull upward, then make a small fanfold in sheet. *Comments:*	☐	☐	☐	
16. Remove soiled pillowcase. Place clean pillowcase on pillow and place under client's head. *Comments:*	☐	☐	☐	
17. Document procedure and client's condition during procedure. *Comments:*	☐	☐	☐	
18. Wash hands/hand hygiene. *Comments:*	☐	☐	☐	

Checklist for Procedure 29-11   Perineal and Genital Care

Name _____ Date _____

School _____

Instructor _____

Course _____

Procedure 29-11 Perineal and Genital Care	Able to Perform	Able to Perform with Assistance	Unable to Perform	Initials/Date
1. Wash hands/hand hygiene, and wear gloves. Gather equipment. Wear other protective equipment, as needed. *Comments:*	☐	☐	☐	
2. Close privacy curtain or door. *Comments:*	☐	☐	☐	
3. Position client. *Comments:*	☐	☐	☐	
4. Place waterproof pads under client in bed or under bedpan, if used. *Comments:*	☐	☐	☐	
5. Removal fecal debris with disposable paper and dispose in toilet. *Comments:*	☐	☐	☐	
6. Spray perineum with washing solution, if indicated. Alternatively, plain water can be used. *Comments:*	☐	☐	☐	
7. Cleanse perineum with wet washcloths (front to back on females), changing to clean area on washcloth with each wipe. Cleanse penis. *Comments:*	☐	☐	☐	

continued on the following page

continued from the previous page

Procedure 29-11 Perineal and Genital Care	Able to Perform	Able to Perform with Assistance	Unable to Perform	Initials/Date
8. Carefully examine gluteal and scrotal folds for debris. Gently examine vulva for debris. *Comments:*	☐	☐	☐	
9. If soap is used, spray area with clean water from the peri-bottle. *Comments:*	☐	☐	☐	
10. Change gloves. *Comments:*	☐	☐	☐	
11. Dry perineum carefully with towel. *Comments:*	☐	☐	☐	
12. If indicated, apply barrier lotion or ointment. *Comments:*	☐	☐	☐	
13. Reposition or dress client, as appropriate. *Comments:*	☐	☐	☐	
14. Dispose of linens and garbage according to hospital policy. *Comments:*	☐	☐	☐	
15. Wash hands/hand hygiene. *Comments:*	☐	☐	☐	
16. Deodorize room, if appropriate. *Comments:*	☐	☐	☐	

Checklist for Procedure 29-12   Oral Care

Name _____   Date _____

School _____

Instructor _____

Course _____

Procedure 29-12 Oral Care	Able to Perform	Able to Perform with Assistance	Unable to Perform	Initials/Date
Self-Care Client: Flossing and Brushing 1. Assemble articles for flossing and brushing. *Comments:*	☐	☐	☐	
2. Provide privacy. *Comments:*	☐	☐	☐	
3. Place client in a high Fowler's position. *Comments:*	☐	☐	☐	
4. Wash hands/hand hygiene, apply gloves. *Comments:*	☐	☐	☐	
5. Arrange articles within client's reach. *Comments:*	☐	☐	☐	
6. Assist client with flossing and brushing, as necessary. Position mirror, emesis basin, and water with straw near client, and place a towel across client's chest. *Comments:*	☐	☐	☐	
7. Assist client with rinsing mouth. *Comments:*	☐	☐	☐	
8. Reposition client, raise side rails, and place call button within reach. *Comments:*	☐	☐	☐	

continued on the following page

continued from the previous page

Procedure 29-12 Oral Care	Able to Perform	Able to Perform with Assistance	Unable to Perform	Initials/Date
9. Rinse, dry, and return articles to proper place. *Comments:*	☐	☐	☐	
10. Remove gloves, wash hands/hand hygiene, and document care. *Comments:*	☐	☐	☐	
Self-Care Client: Denture Care 11. Assemble articles for denture cleaning. *Comments:*	☐	☐	☐	
12. Provide privacy. *Comments:*	☐	☐	☐	
13. Assist client to a high Fowler's position. *Comments:*	☐	☐	☐	
14. Wash hands/hands hygiene, and apply gloves. *Comments:*	☐	☐	☐	
15. Assist client with denture removal of top and bottom denture. Place in denture cup. *Comments:*	☐	☐	☐	
16. Apply toothpaste to brush, and brush dentures either with cool water in emesis basin or under running water in sink. Pad sink with towel to protect dentures in case dropped. *Comments:*	☐	☐	☐	

continued on the following page

continued from the previous page

Procedure 29-12 Oral Care	Able to Perform	Able to Perform with Assistance	Unable to Perform	Initials/Date
17. Rinse thoroughly. *Comments:*	☐	☐	☐	
18. Assist client with rinsing mouth and replacing dentures. *Comments:*	☐	☐	☐	
19. Reposition client with side rails up and call button within reach. *Comments:*	☐	☐	☐	
20. Rinse, dry, and return articles to proper place. *Comments:*	☐	☐	☐	
21. Remove gloves, wash hands/hand hygiene, and document care. *Comments:*	☐	☐	☐	
Full-Care Client: Brushing and Flossing 22. Assemble articles for flossing and brushing. *Comments:*	☐	☐	☐	
23. Provide privacy. *Comments:*	☐	☐	☐	
24. Wash hands/hand hygiene, and apply gloves. *Comments:*	☐	☐	☐	
25. Position client as condition allows. *Comments:*	☐	☐	☐	

continued on the following page

continued from the previous page

Procedure 29-12 Oral Care	Able to Perform	Able to Perform with Assistance	Unable to Perform	Initials/Date
26. Place towel across client's chest or under face and mouth if head is turned to one side. *Comments:*	☐	☐	☐	
27. Moisten toothbrush or toothette, apply small amount of toothpaste, and brush teeth and gums. *Comments:*	☐	☐	☐	
28. Grasp dental floss in both hands or use a floss holder and floss between all teeth; hold floss against tooth while moving floss up and down sides of teeth. *Comments:*	☐	☐	☐	
29. Assist client in rinsing mouth. *Comments:*	☐	☐	☐	
30. Reapply toothpaste and brush the teeth and gums using friction in a vertical or circular motion. Brush all surfaces from every angle. *Comments:*	☐	☐	☐	
31. Assist client in rinsing and drying mouth. *Comments:*	☐	☐	☐	
32. Apply lip moisturizer, if appropriate. *Comments:*	☐	☐	☐	
33. Reposition client, raise side rails, and place call button within reach. *Comments:*	☐	☐	☐	

continued on the following page

continued from the previous page

Procedure 29-12 Oral Care	Able to Perform	Able to Perform with Assistance	Unable to Perform	Initials/Date
34. Rinse, dry, and return articles to proper place. *Comments:*	☐	☐	☐	
35. Remove gloves, wash hands/hand hygiene, and document care. *Comments:*	☐	☐	☐	
Clients at Risk for or with an Alteration of the Oral Cavity 36. Assemble articles for flossing and brushing. *Comments:*	☐	☐	☐	
37. Provide privacy. *Comments:*	☐	☐	☐	
38. Wash hands/hand hygiene, and apply gloves. *Comments:*	☐	☐	☐	
39. Bleeding: a. Assess oral cavity for signs of bleeding. b. Proceed with oral care, except: • Do not floss. • Use a soft toothbrush, toothette, or a tongue blade padded with 3 × 3 gauze sponges to gently swab teeth and gums. • Dispose of padded tongue blade into a biohazard bag, according to institutional policy. • Rinse with tepid water. *Comments:*	☐	☐	☐	

continued on the following page

continued from the previous page

Procedure 29-12 Oral Care	Able to Perform	Able to Perform with Assistance	Unable to Perform	Initials/Date

40. Infection:
  a. Assess oral cavity for signs of bleeding.
  b. Culture lesions, as ordered.
  c. Proceed with actions for oral care for a full-care client, except:
    • Do not floss.
    • Use prescribed antiseptic solution.
    • Use a tongue blade padded with 3 × 3 gauze sponges to gently swab teeth and gums.
    • Dispose of padded tongue blade into a biohazard bag, according to institutional policy.
    • Rinse mouth with tepid water.
    • Apply additional solution as prescribed.
Comments:
	☐	☐	☐	

41. Ulceration:
  a. Assess oral cavity with a padded tongue blade and flashlight for signs of ulceration.
  b. Culture lesions, as ordered.
  c. Proceed with the actions for oral care for a full-care client, except:
    • Do not floss.
    • Use prescribed antiseptic solution.
    • Use a tongue blade padded with 3 × 3 gauze sponges to gently swab teeth and gums.
    • Dispose of padded tongue blade into a biohazard bag, according to institutional policy.
    • Rinse mouth with tepid water.
    • Apply additional solution, as prescribed.
Comments:
	☐	☐	☐	

Unconscious (Comatose) Client 42. Assemble articles for flossing and brushing. *Comments:*	☐	☐	☐	

continued on the following page

continued from the previous page

Procedure 29-12 Oral Care	Able to Perform	Able to Perform with Assistance	Unable to Perform	Initials/Date
43. Provide privacy. *Comments:*	☐	☐	☐	
44. Wash hands/hand hygiene, and apply gloves. *Comments:*	☐	☐	☐	
45. Explain procedure to client. *Comments:*	☐	☐	☐	
46. Place client in a lateral position, with head turned toward side. *Comments:*	☐	☐	☐	
47. Using a floss holder, floss between all teeth. *Comments:*	☐	☐	☐	
48. Moisten toothbrush or toothette, and brush teeth and gums, using friction in a vertical or circular motion. Do not use toothpaste. All surfaces of teeth should be brushed from every angle. *Comments:*	☐	☐	☐	
49. After flossing and brushing, rinse mouth with an Asepto syringe and perform oral suction. *Comments:*	☐	☐	☐	
50. Dry client's mouth. *Comments:*	☐	☐	☐	

continued on the following page

continued from the previous page

Procedure 29-12 Oral Care	Able to Perform	Able to Perform with Assistance	Unable to Perform	Initials/Date
51. Apply lip moisturizer. *Comments:*	☐	☐	☐	
52. Leave client in a lateral position with head turned toward side for 30–60 minutes after oral hygiene care. Suction 1 more time. Remove towel from under client's mouth and face. *Comments:*	☐	☐	☐	
53. Dispose of any contaminated items in a biohazard bag and clean, dry, and return all articles to appropriate place. *Comments:*	☐	☐	☐	
54. Remove gloves, wash hands/hand hygiene, and document care. *Comments:*	☐	☐	☐	

Checklist for Procedure 29-13 Eye Care

Name _____ Date _____

School _____

Instructor _____

Course _____

Procedure 29-13 Eye Care	Able to Perform	Able to Perform with Assistance	Unable to Perform	Initials/Date
Artificial Eye Removal 1. Inquire about client's care regimen and gather equipment accordingly. *Comments:*	☐	☐	☐	
2. Provide privacy. *Comments:*	☐	☐	☐	
3. Wash hands/hand hygiene, and apply gloves. *Comments:*	☐	☐	☐	
4. Place client in a semi-Fowler's position. *Comments:*	☐	☐	☐	
5. Place cotton balls in emesis basin filled halfway with warm tap water. *Comments:*	☐	☐	☐	
6. Place 3 × 3 gauze sponges in bottom of second emesis basin and fill halfway with mild soap and tepid water. *Comments:*	☐	☐	☐	

continued on the following page

continued from the previous page

Procedure 29-13 Eye Care	Able to Perform	Able to Perform with Assistance	Unable to Perform	Initials/Date
7. Grasp and squeeze excess water from a cotton ball. Cleanse eyelid with moistened cotton ball, starting at inner canthus and moving outward toward outer canthus. After each use, dispose of cotton ball in biohazard bag. Repeat procedure until eyelid is clean (without dried secretions). *Comments:*	☐	☐	☐	
8. Remove artificial eye: a. Using dominant hand, raise client's upper eyelid with index finger, and depress lower eyelid with thumb. b. Cup nondominant hand under client's lower eyelid. c. Apply slight pressure with index finger between brow and artificial eye, and remove it. Place eye in emesis basin filled with warm, soapy water. *Comments:*	☐	☐	☐	
9. Grasp a moistened cotton ball and cleanse around edge of eye socket. Dispose of soiled cotton ball into biohazard bag. *Comments:*	☐	☐	☐	
10. Inspect eye socket for any signs of irritation, drainage, or crusting. *Comments:*	☐	☐	☐	
11. Eye socket irrigation (if needed): a. Lower head of bed and place client in supine position. Place protector pad on bed. Turn head toward socket side and slightly extend neck.	☐	☐	☐	

continued on the following page

continued from the previous page

Procedure 29-13 Eye Care	Able to Perform	Able to Perform with Assistance	Unable to Perform	Initials/Date
b. Fill irrigation syringe with prescribed amount and type of irrigating solution. c. With nondominant hand, separate eyelids with forefinger and thumb while resting fingers on the brow and cheekbone. d. Hold irrigating syringe in dominant hand several inches above inner canthus; gently apply pressure on plunger, directing flow of solution from inner canthus along conjunctival sac. e. Irrigate until prescribed amount of solution has been used. f. Wipe eyelids with moistened cotton ball after irrigating. Dispose in biohazard bag. g. Pat skin dry with towel. h. Return client to semi-Fowler's position. i. Remove gloves, wash hands/hand hygiene, and apply clean gloves. *Comments:*				
12. Clean artificial eye in basin of warm, soapy water. *Comments:*	☐	☐	☐	
13. Rinse the prosthesis under running water or place in the clean basin of tepid water. Do not dry the prosthesis. *Note:* Either reinsert prosthesis (Action 14) or store in a container (Action 15). *Comments:*	☐	☐	☐	
14. Reinsert prosthesis: a. With the thumb of nondominant hand, raise and hold upper eyelid open.	☐	☐	☐	

continued on the following page

continued from the previous page

Procedure 29-13 Eye Care	Able to Perform	Able to Perform with Assistance	Unable to Perform	Initials/Date
b. With dominant hand, grasp artificial eye so indented part is facing toward client's nose and slide it under upper eyelid as far as possible c. Depress lower lid. d. Pull lower lid forward to cover edge of prosthesis. *Comments:*				
15. Place cleaned artificial eye in a labeled container with saline or tap water solution. *Comments:*	☐	☐	☐	
16. Grasp moistened cotton ball and squeeze out excessive moisture. Wipe eyelid from inner to outer canthus. Dispose in a biohazard bag. *Comments:*	☐	☐	☐	
17. Clean, dry, and replace equipment. *Comments:*	☐	☐	☐	
18. Reposition client, raise side rails, and place call button within reach. *Comments:*	☐	☐	☐	
19. Dispose of biohazard bag according to institutional policy. *Comments:*	☐	☐	☐	
20. Remove gloves. Wash hands/hand hygiene. *Comments:*	☐	☐	☐	

continued on the following page

continued from the previous page

Procedure 29-13 Eye Care	Able to Perform	Able to Perform with Assistance	Unable to Perform	Initials/Date
21. Document procedure, client's response and participation, and client teaching and level of understanding. *Comments:*	☐	☐	☐	
Contact Lens Removal 22. Assemble equipment for lens removal. *Comments:*	☐	☐	☐	
23. Assess level of assistance needed, provide privacy, and explain procedure to client. *Comments:*	☐	☐	☐	
24. Wash hands/hand hygiene. *Comments:*	☐	☐	☐	
25. Assist client to a semi-Fowler's position, if needed. *Comments:*	☐	☐	☐	
26. Drape a clean towel over client's chest. *Comments:*	☐	☐	☐	
27. Prepare lens storage case with prescribed solution. *Comments:*	☐	☐	☐	
28. Instruct client to look straight ahead. Assess location of lens. If it is not on cornea, either you or client gently move lens toward cornea with pad of index finger. *Comments:*	☐	☐	☐	

continued on the following page

continued from the previous page

Procedure 29-13 Eye Care	Able to Perform	Able to Perform with Assistance	Unable to Perform	Initials/Date

29. Remove lens.
  a. Hard lens:
    • Cup nondominant hand under eye.
    • Gently place index finger on outside corner of eye and pull toward temple and ask client to blink. Catch lens in nondominant hand.
  b. Soft lens:
    • With nondominant hand, separate eyelid with thumb and middle finger.
    • With index finger of dominant hand gently placed on lower edge of lens, slide lens downward onto sclera and gently squeeze the lens.
    • Release top eyelid (continue holding lower lid down) and remove lens with your index finger and thumb.
Note: If Action 29 is unsuccessful, secure a suction cup to remove the contact lens. If unable to remove the lens, notify the physician or qualified practitioner.
Comments:
	☐	☐	☐	

30. Store lens in correct compartment of the case ("right" or "left"). Label with client's name. *Comments:*	☐	☐	☐	
31. Remove and store other lens by repeating Actions 29 and 30. *Comments:*	☐	☐	☐	
32. Assess eyes for irritation or redness. *Comments:*	☐	☐	☐	

continued on the following page

continued from the previous page

Procedure 29-13 Eye Care	Able to Perform	Able to Perform with Assistance	Unable to Perform	Initials/Date
33. Store lens case in safe place. *Comments:*	☐	☐	☐	
34. Dispose of soiled articles, and clean and return reusable articles to proper location. *Comments:*	☐	☐	☐	
35. Reposition client, raise side rails, and place call light in reach. *Comments:*	☐	☐	☐	
36. Remove gloves. Wash hands/hand hygiene. *Comments:*	☐	☐	☐	
37. Document procedure, client's response and assessment findings, and lenses storage place. *Comments:*	☐	☐	☐	

Checklist for Procedure 30-1   Medication Administration: Oral, Sublingual, and Buccal

Name _____ Date _____

School _____

Instructor _____

Course _____

Procedure 30-1 Medication Administration: Oral, Sublingual, and Buccal	Able to Perform	Able to Perform with Assistance	Unable to Perform	Initials/Date
1. Wash hands/hand hygiene, and apply clean gloves. *Comments:*	☐	☐	☐	
2. Arrange medication tray or cart. Follow institutional protocol. *Comments:*	☐	☐	☐	
3. Unlock medication cart or log on to computer. *Comments:*	☐	☐	☐	
4. Prepare medication for one client at a time following five rights. Select correct drug from medication drawer according to the MAR. Calculate drug dosage, if needed. *Comments:*	☐	☐	☐	
5. To prepare a tablet or capsule: Pour required number of tablets or capsules into bottle cap and transfer medication to a medication cup without touching. • Scored tablets may be broken. • A unit-dose tablet should be placed directly into medicine cup *without* opening until administered.	☐	☐	☐	

continued on the following page

continued from the previous page

Procedure 30-1 Medication Administration: Oral, Sublingual, and Buccal	Able to Perform	Able to Perform with Assistance	Unable to Perform	Initials/Date
• For clients with difficulty swallowing, some tablets can be crushed into a powder using a mortar and pestle or by being placed between two paper medication cups and ground with a blunt object, then mixed in a small amount of applesauce or custard. Time-released or specially coated medications must not be crushed. Check with pharmacy if uncertain. *Comments:*				
6. To prepare a liquid medication: Remove bottle cap from container and place cap upside down on cart. Hold bottle with label up and medication cup at eye level while pouring. Fill cup to desired level using surface or base of the meniscus as scale, not edge of liquid on cup. Wipe lip of bottle with paper towel. *Comments:*	☐	☐	☐	
7. To prepare narcotic: Obtain key to narcotic drawer and check narcotic record for drug count when signing out dose. If drug count does not agree with records, report to charge nurse immediately. Institution may require filing of an incident report. *Comments:*	☐	☐	☐	
8. Check expiration date on all medications. • Double-check MAR with prepared drugs. • Return stock medications to shelf or drawer. • Place MARs with client's medications. • Do not leave drugs unattended. *Comments:*	☐	☐	☐	

continued on the following page

continued from the previous page

Procedure 30-1 Medication Administration: Oral, Sublingual, and Buccal	Able to Perform	Able to Perform with Assistance	Unable to Perform	Initials/Date
9. Administer medications to client: Observe the correct time to give medication. • Identify client by reading client's name bracelet, repeating name, and asking client to state name. Additionally, check hospital number if name alert or client is not reliable. • Check drug packaging if present to ensure medication type and dosage. • Assess client's condition and form of medication. • Perform any assessment, such as pulse or blood pressure, required for specific medications. • Explain purpose of drug and ask if client has any questions. • Assist client to sitting or lateral position. • Allow client to hold tablet or medication cup. • Give glass of water or other liquid, and straw, if needed, to help client swallow medication. • For *sublingual* medications, instruct client to place medication under tongue and allow to dissolve completely. • For *buccal* administration of drugs, instruct client to place medication in mouth against cheek until it dissolves completely. • For *oral* medications given through a *nasogastric tube*, crush tablets or open capsules and dissolve powder with 20–30 ml of warm water in a cup. Be sure medication will still be properly absorbed if crushed and dissolved. Check placement of feeding tube or nasogastric tube before instilling anything but air into tube. • Remain with client until each medication has been swallowed or dissolved. • Assist client into comfortable position. *Comments:*	☐	☐	☐	

continued on the following page

continued from the previous page

Procedure 30-1 Medication Administration: Oral, Sublingual, and Buccal	Able to Perform	Able to Perform with Assistance	Unable to Perform	Initials/Date
10. Dispose of soiled supplies. Wash hands/ hand hygiene. *Comments:*	☐	☐	☐	
11. Record time and route of administration on MAR and return it to client's file. *Comments:*	☐	☐	☐	
12. Return cart to medicine room; restock supplies, as needed. Clean work area. *Comments:*	☐	☐	☐	

Checklist for Procedure 30-2   Withdrawing Medication from an Ampule

Name _____ Date _____

School _____

Instructor _____

Course _____

Procedure 30-2 Withdrawing Medication from an Ampule	Able to Perform	Able to Perform with Assistance	Unable to Perform	Initials/Date
1. Wash hands/hand hygiene, and secure supplies. *Comments:*	☐	☐	☐	
2. Select appropriate ampule. *Comments:*	☐	☐	☐	
3. Select syringe with filter needle. *Comments:*	☐	☐	☐	
4. Obtain a sterile gauze pad. *Comments:*	☐	☐	☐	
5. Select and set aside appropriate length of safety needle for planned injection. *Comments:*	☐	☐	☐	
6. Clear a workspace. *Comments:*	☐	☐	☐	
7. Observe ampule for location of medication. *Comments:*	☐	☐	☐	
8. If medication is trapped in top, flick neck of ampule repeatedly with fingernail while holding ampule upright. *Comments:*	☐	☐	☐	

continued on the following page

continued from the previous page

Procedure 30-2 **Withdrawing Medication from an Ampule**	**Able to Perform**	**Able to Perform with Assistance**	**Unable to Perform**	**Initials/Date**
9. Wrap sterile gauze pad around neck and snap off top in an outward motion directed away from self. *Comments:*	☐	☐	☐	
10. Invert ampule and place needle into liquid. Gently withdraw medication into syringe. *Comments:*	☐	☐	☐	
11. Alternately, place ampule on counter, hold and tilt slightly with nondominant hand. Insert needle below level of liquid and gently draw liquid into syringe, tilting ampule, as needed, to reach all liquid. *Comments:*	☐	☐	☐	
12. Remove filter needle and replace with safety injection needle. *Comments:*	☐	☐	☐	
13. Dispose of filter needle and glass ampule (including lid) in appropriate sharps container. *Comments:*	☐	☐	☐	
14. Label syringe with drug, dose, date, and time. *Comments:*	☐	☐	☐	
15. Wash hands/hand hygiene. *Comments:*	☐	☐	☐	

Checklist for Procedure 30-3   Withdrawing Medication from a Vial

Name _____ Date _____

School _____

Instructor _____

Course _____

Procedure 30-3 Withdrawing Medication from a Vial	Able to Perform	Able to Perform with Assistance	Unable to Perform	Initials/Date
1. Wash hands/hand hygiene; secure supplies and apply gloves (optional). *Comments:*	☐	☐	☐	
2. Select appropriate vial. *Comments:*	☐	☐	☐	
3. Verify prescribing practitioner's orders. *Comments:*	☐	☐	☐	
4. Check expiration date. *Comments:*	☐	☐	☐	
5. Determine route of medication delivery and select appropriate size syringe and needle. *Comments:*	☐	☐	☐	
6. While holding syringe at eye level, withdraw plunger to desired volume of medication. *Comments:*	☐	☐	☐	
7. Clean rubber top of vial with a 70% alcohol pad. *Comments:*	☐	☐	☐	
8. Using sterile technique, uncap needle. *Comments:*	☐	☐	☐	

continued on the following page

continued from the previous page

Procedure 30-3 Withdrawing Medication from a Vial	Able to Perform	Able to Perform with Assistance	Unable to Perform	Initials/Date
9. Lay needle cap on clean surface. *Comments:*	☐	☐	☐	
10. Placing needle in center of vial, inject air slowly. Do not cause turbulence. *Comments:*	☐	☐	☐	
11. Invert vial and slowly, using gentle negative pressure, withdraw medication. Keep needle tip in liquid. *Comments:*	☐	☐	☐	
12. With syringe at eye level, determine appropriate dose has been reached by volume. *Comments:*	☐	☐	☐	
13. Slowly withdraw needle from vial. Follow institution's policy regarding recapping and changing needles. *Comments:*	☐	☐	☐	
14. Using ink, mark current date and time and initials on vial. *Comments:*	☐	☐	☐	
15. Label syringe with drug, dose, date, and time. *Comments:*	☐	☐	☐	
16. Wash hands/hand hygiene. *Comments:*	☐	☐	☐	

Checklist for Procedure 30-4 Mixing Medications from Two Vials into One Syringe

Name _____ Date _____

School _____

Instructor _____

Course _____

Procedure 30-4 Mixing Medications from Two Vials into One Syringe	Able to Perform	Able to Perform with Assistance	Unable to Perform	Initials/Date
1. Check MAR against prescribing practitioner's written orders. *Comments:*	☐	☐	☐	
2. Check for drug allergies. *Comments:*	☐	☐	☐	
3. Wash hands/hand hygiene. *Comments:*	☐	☐	☐	
4. Gather equipment needed. Prepare medication for one client at a time. *Comments:*	☐	☐	☐	
5. Check need for one medication to be drawn up before other. *Comments:*	☐	☐	☐	
6. Determine total medication volume (in milliliters) in syringe after drawing both medications into syringe. *Comments:*	☐	☐	☐	
7. Swab top of each vial with alcohol. *Comments:*	☐	☐	☐	

continued on the following page

continued from the previous page

Procedure 30-4 Mixing Medications from Two Vials into One Syringe	Able to Perform	Able to Perform with Assistance	Unable to Perform	Initials/Date
8. Draw air into syringe equal to amount of medication to be drawn up from second vial. Inject air into second vial and remove syringe and needle from vial. Some protocols require changing needles. *Comments:*	☐	☐	☐	
9. Draw air into syringe equal to amount of medication to be drawn up from first vial. Inject air into first vial. Keep needle and syringe in vial. *Comments:*	☐	☐	☐	
10. Pulling back on plunger, withdraw correct amount (in milliliters) of medication from first vial. *Comments:*	☐	☐	☐	
11. Remove syringe from first vial and insert it into second vial. Withdraw medication from second vial to volume (in milliliters) total of both medications summed together. *Comments:*	☐	☐	☐	
12. Either leave needle in second vial until just before injecting medication or follow institution's policy regarding recapping needles. *Comments:*	☐	☐	☐	
13. Wash hands/hand hygiene. *Comments:*	☐	☐	☐	

continued on the following page

continued from the previous page

Procedure 30-4 Mixing Medications from Two Vials into One Syringe	Able to Perform	Able to Perform with Assistance	Unable to Perform	Initials/Date
Mixing Insulin The clear insulin (regular, short-acting) is drawn up first, then cloudy solution (intermediate or long-acting). Check manufacturer's information regarding types of insulin and carefully assess response of client. Before administering insulin, dosage must be double-checked by two professionals. An inaccurate dose of insulin can be life-threatening. 1. Check client's most recent blood glucose level, dietary intake, oral intake status (e.g., is NPO) and signs and symptoms related to glucose level. *Comments:*	☐	☐	☐	
2. Repeat Actions 1–4 above. *Comments:*	☐	☐	☐	
3. Remove caps from insulin vials (if necessary). Gently rotate (never shake) suspension insulin (e.g., NPH, intermediate, or long-acting insulin) until no sediment is at bottom of vial. *Comments:*	☐	☐	☐	
4. Wipe off insulin vials' tops with alcohol sponge. *Comments:*	☐	☐	☐	
5. Draw back air into syringe equal to total dose of both insulin solutions. Insert needle and syringe into vial with cloudy, suspension (intermediate or long-acting insulin) and inject air equal to amount to be given of that insulin. Do not touch solution with needle. *Comments:*	☐	☐	☐	

continued on the following page

continued from the previous page

Procedure 30-4 **Mixing Medications from Two Vials into One Syringe**	**Able to Perform**	**Able to Perform with Assistance**	**Unable to Perform**	**Initials/Date**
6. Insert needle and syringe into vial of short-acting or regular insulin and inject air equal to amount to be given. *Comments:*	☐	☐	☐	
7. Keep needle and syringe in solution. Invert vial and withdraw medication slowly and accurately. *Comments:*	☐	☐	☐	
8. Withdraw needle and expel any air bubbles and check dose with another nurse. *Comments:*	☐	☐	☐	
9. Invert vial with longer-acting insulin, holding plunger carefully, and withdraw long-acting insulin, being careful not to inject any regular insulin into vial. Check dose with another nurse. *Comments:*	☐	☐	☐	
10. Store insulin properly according to manufacturer's specifications. *Comments:*	☐	☐	☐	
11. Wash hands/hand hygiene; prepare to administer injection. *Comments:*	☐	☐	☐	

Checklist for Procedure 30-5   Medication Administration: Intradermal

Name _____   Date _____

School _____

Instructor _____

Course _____

Procedure 30-5 Medication Administration: Intradermal	Able to Perform	Able to Perform with Assistance	Unable to Perform	Initials/Date
1. Wash hands/hand hygiene; apply clean gloves. *Comments:*	☐	☐	☐	
2. Provide privacy. Identify client. *Comments:*	☐	☐	☐	
3. Select injection site. *Comments:*	☐	☐	☐	
4. Select 1/4- to 5/8-inch 25–27 gauge needle. *Comments:*	☐	☐	☐	
5. Assist client into a comfortable position. Distract client by talking about an interesting subject. *Comments:*	☐	☐	☐	
6. Use antiseptic swab in a circular motion to clean skin at site. *Comments:*	☐	☐	☐	
7. While holding swab between fingers of nondominant hand, pull cap from needle. *Comments:*	☐	☐	☐	

continued on the following page

continued from the previous page

Procedure 30-5 Medication Administration: Intradermal	Able to Perform	Able to Perform with Assistance	Unable to Perform	Initials/Date
8. Administer injection: • With nondominant hand, stretch skin over site with forefinger and thumb. • Insert needle slowly at a 5° to 15° angle, bevel up, until resistance is felt; then advance to no more than 1/8 inch below skin. Needle tip should be seen through skin. • Slow inject medication. Resistance will be felt. • Note a small bleb forming under skin surface. *Comments:*	☐	☐	☐	
9. Withdraw needle while applying gentle pressure with antiseptic swab. *Comments:*	☐	☐	☐	
10. Do not massage site. *Comments:*	☐	☐	☐	
11. Assist client to comfortable position. *Comments:*	☐	☐	☐	
12. Discard uncapped needle and syringe in safe receptacle. *Comments:*	☐	☐	☐	
13. Remove gloves; wash hands/hand hygiene. *Comments:*	☐	☐	☐	

Checklist for Procedure 30-6   Medication Administration: Subcutaneous

Name _____   Date _____

School _____

Instructor _____

Course _____

Procedure 30-6 Medication Administration: Subcutaneous	Able to Perform	Able to Perform with Assistance	Unable to Perform	Initials/Date
1. Wash hands/hand hygiene; apply clean gloves. Select appropriate syringe for medication being given. *Comments:*	☐	☐	☐	
2. Provide privacy. Identify client. *Comments:*	☐	☐	☐	
3. Select injection site. *Comments:*	☐	☐	☐	
4. Select needle size. *Comments:*	☐	☐	☐	
5. Assist client into a comfortable position. *Comments:*	☐	☐	☐	
6. Use antiseptic swab to clean skin at site. *Comments:*	☐	☐	☐	
7. While holding swab between fingers of nondominant hand, pull cap from needle. *Comments:*	☐	☐	☐	
8. Administer injection: • Hold syringe between thumb and forefinger of dominant hand like a dart. • Pinch skin with nondominant hand. • Inject needle quickly and firmly (like a dart) at a 45° to 90° angle.	☐	☐	☐	

continued on the following page

continued from the previous page

Procedure 30-6 Medication Administration: Subcutaneous	Able to Perform	Able to Perform with Assistance	Unable to Perform	Initials/Date
• Release skin. • Grasp lower end of syringe with nondominant hand and position dominant hand to end of plunger. Do not move syringe. • Pull back on plunger to ascertain that needle is not in a vein. If no blood appears, slowly inject medication. (Aspiration is contraindicated with some medications; check with the pharmacy if unclear.) *Comments:*				
9. Remove hand from injection site and quickly withdraw needle. Apply pressure with antiseptic swab. *Comments:*	☐	☐	☐	
10. Some medications should not be massaged. Ask pharmacy if unclear. *Comments:*	☐	☐	☐	
11. Assist client to a comfortable position. *Comments:*	☐	☐	☐	
12. Discard uncapped needle and syringe in disposable needle receptacle. *Comments:*	☐	☐	☐	
13. Remove gloves; wash hands/hand hygiene. *Comments:*	☐	☐	☐	

Checklist for Procedure 30-7   Medication Administration: Intramuscular

Name _____ Date _____

School _____

Instructor _____

Course _____

Procedure 30-7 Medication Administration: Intramuscular	Able to Perform	Able to Perform with Assistance	Unable to Perform	Initials/Date
1. Wash hands/hand hygiene; put on clean gloves. *Comments:*	☐	☐	☐	
2. Close door or curtains around bed and keep gown or sheet draped over client. Identify client. *Comments:*	☐	☐	☐	
3. Select injection site. *Comments:*	☐	☐	☐	
4. Select needle size. *Comments:*	☐	☐	☐	
5. Assist client into a comfortable position. Consider injection site. *Comments:*	☐	☐	☐	
6. Use antiseptic swab to clean skin at site. *Comments:*	☐	☐	☐	
7. While holding swab between fingers of nondominant hand, pull cap from needle. *Comments:*	☐	☐	☐	
8. Administer injection: • Hold syringe between thumb and forefinger of dominant hand like a dart.	☐	☐	☐	

continued on the following page

continued from the previous page

Procedure 30-7 Medication Administration: Intramuscular	Able to Perform	Able to Perform with Assistance	Unable to Perform	Initials/Date
• Spread skin tightly or pinch a generous section of tissue firmly—for cachectic patients. • Inject needle quickly and firmly (like a dart) at a 90° angle. • Release skin. • Grasp lower end of syringe with nondominant hand and position dominant hand to end of plunger. Do not move syringe. • Pull back on plunger and aspirate to ascertain if needle is in vein. If no blood appears, slowly inject medication. *Comments:*				
9. Remove nondominant hand and quickly withdraw needle. Apply pressure with antiseptic swab. *Comments:*	☐	☐	☐	
10. Apply pressure. Certain protocols suggest gentle massaging action. *Comments:*	☐	☐	☐	
11. Assist client to a comfortable position. *Comments:*	☐	☐	☐	
12. Discard uncapped needle and syringe in specified biohazard sharps container. *Comments:*	☐	☐	☐	
13. Remove gloves; wash hands/hand hygiene. *Comments:*	☐	☐	☐	

Checklist for Procedure 30-8   Medication Administration: Secondary Administration Sets (Piggyback)

Name _____   Date _____

School _____

Instructor _____

Course _____

Procedure 30-8 Medication Administration: Secondary Administration Sets (Piggyback)	Able to Perform	Able to Perform with Assistance	Unable to Perform	Initials/Date
1. Check prescribing practitioner's orders. *Comments:*	☐	☐	☐	
2. Wash hands/hand hygiene. Gloves are not necessary if adding fluids to an existing infusion line. Secure IV tubing for piggyback administration. *Comments:*	☐	☐	☐	
3. Check client's identification bracelet. *Comments:*	☐	☐	☐	
4. Explain procedure and reason drug is being given. *Comments:*	☐	☐	☐	
5. Prepare medication bag: • Close clamp on tubing of infusion set. • Spike medication bag with infusion tubing. • Open clamp. • Allow tubing to be filled with solution to evacuate air from tubing. *Comments:*	☐	☐	☐	
6. Hang piggyback medication bag above level of primary IV bag. *Comments:*	☐	☐	☐	

continued on the following page

continued from the previous page

Procedure 30-8 **Medication Administration: Secondary Administration Sets (Piggyback)**	**Able to Perform**	**Able to Perform with Assistance**	**Unable to Perform**	**Initials/Date**
7. Connect piggyback tubing to primary tubing at Y-port: • For needleless system, remove cap on port and connect tubing. • If a needle is used, clean port with antiseptic swab and insert small-gauge needle into center of port. • Secure tubing with adhesive tape. *Comments:*	☐	☐	☐	
8. Administer medication: • Check prescribed length of time for infusion. • Regulate flow rate of piggyback by adjusting regulator clamp. • Observe whether backflow valve on piggyback has stopped flow of primary infusion during drug administration. *Comments:*	☐	☐	☐	
9. Check primary infusion line when medication is finished: • Regulate primary infusion rate. • Leave secondary bag and tubing in place for next drug administration. *Comments:*	☐	☐	☐	
10. Dispose of all used materials and place needles in needle biohazard sharps container. *Comments:*	☐	☐	☐	
11. Wash hands/hand hygiene. *Comments:*	☐	☐	☐	

Checklist for Procedure 30-9   Medication Administration: Eye and Ear

Name _____ Date _____

School _____

Instructor _____

Course _____

Procedure 30-9 Medication Administration: Eye and Ear	Able to Perform	Able to Perform with Assistance	Unable to Perform	Initials/Date
Eye Medication 1. Check for allergies or contraindications. *Comments:*	☐	☐	☐	
2. Gather necessary equipment. *Comments:*	☐	☐	☐	
3. Follow five rights of drug administration. *Comments:*	☐	☐	☐	
4. Take medication to client's room and place on a clean surface. *Comments:*	☐	☐	☐	
5. Check client's identification armband. *Comments:*	☐	☐	☐	
6. Explain procedure to client. *Comments:*	☐	☐	☐	
7. Wash hands/hand hygiene; apply nonsterile, latex-free gloves, if needed. *Comments:*	☐	☐	☐	
8. Place client in supine position with head slightly hyperextended. *Comments:*	☐	☐	☐	

continued on the following page

continued from the previous page

Procedure 30-9 Medication Administration: Eye and Ear	Able to Perform	Able to Perform with Assistance	Unable to Perform	Initials/Date
Instilling Eye Drops 9. Remove cap from eye bottle and place cap on its side. *Comments:*	☐	☐	☐	
10. Squeeze prescribed amount of medication into eyedropper. *Comments:*	☐	☐	☐	
11. Place a tissue below lower lid. *Comments:*	☐	☐	☐	
12. With dominant hand, hold eyedropper 1/2–3/4 inch above eyeball; rest hand on client's forehead to stabilize. *Comments:*	☐	☐	☐	
13. Place hand on cheekbone and expose lower conjunctival sac by pulling down on cheek. *Comments:*	☐	☐	☐	
14. Instruct client to look up and drop prescribed number of drops into center of conjunctival sac. *Comments:*	☐	☐	☐	
15. Instruct client to gently close eyes and move eyes. Briefly place fingers on either side of client's nose to close tear ducts. *Comments:*	☐	☐	☐	
16. Remove gloves; wash hands/hand hygiene. *Comments:*	☐	☐	☐	

continued on the following page

continued from the previous page

Procedure 30-9 Medication Administration: Eye and Ear	Able to Perform	Able to Perform with Assistance	Unable to Perform	Initials/Date
17. Record on MAR route, site (which eye), and time administered. *Comments:*	☐	☐	☐	
Eye Ointment Application 18. Repeat Actions 1–8. *Comments:*	☐	☐	☐	
19. Lower lid: • With nondominant hand, gently separate client's eyelids with thumb and finger and grasp lower lid near margin immediately below lashes; exert pressure downward over bony prominence of cheek. • Instruct client to look up. • Apply eye ointment along inside edge of entire lower eyelid, from inner to outer canthus. *Comments:*	☐	☐	☐	
20. Upper lid: • Instruct client to look down. • With nondominant hand, gently grasp client's lashes near center of upper lid with thumb and index finger, and draw lid up and away from eyeball. • Squeeze ointment along upper lid starting at inner canthus. *Comments:*	☐	☐	☐	
21. Repeat Actions 16 and 17. *Comments:*	☐	☐	☐	
Medication Disk 22. Repeat Actions 1–8. *Comments:*	☐	☐	☐	

continued on the following page

continued from the previous page

Procedure 30-9 Medication Administration: Eye and Ear	Able to Perform	Able to Perform with Assistance	Unable to Perform	Initials/Date
23. Open sterile package and press dominant, sterile gloved finger against oval disk so that it lies lengthwise across fingertip. *Comments:*	☐	☐	☐	
24. Instruct client to look up. *Comments:*	☐	☐	☐	
25. With nondominant hand, gently pull client's lower eyelid down and place disk horizontally in conjunctival sac. • Then pull lower eyelid out, up, and over disk. • Instruct client to blink several times. • If disk is still visible, repeat actions above. • Once disk is in place, instruct client to gently press fingers against closed lids; do not rub eyes or move disk across cornea. • If disk falls out, pick it up, rinse under cool water, and reinsert. *Comments:*	☐	☐	☐	
26. If disk is prescribed for both eyes, repeat Actions 23–25. *Comments:*	☐	☐	☐	
27. Repeat Actions 15–17. *Comments:*	☐	☐	☐	
Removing an Eye Medication Disk 28. Repeat Actions 3 and 5–8. *Comments:*	☐	☐	☐	
29. Remove disk: • With nondominant hand, invert lower eyelid and identify disk.	☐	☐	☐	

continued on the following page

continued from the previous page

Procedure 30-9 Medication Administration: Eye and Ear	Able to Perform	Able to Perform with Assistance	Unable to Perform	Initials/Date
• If disk is located in upper eye, instruct client to close eye, and place your fingers on closed eyelid. Apply gentle, long, circular strokes; instruct client to open eye. Disk should be located in corner of eye. With your fingertip, slide disk to lower lid, and then proceed. • With dominant hand, use forefinger to slide disk onto lid and out of client's eye. *Comments:*				
30. Remove gloves; wash hands/hand hygiene. *Comments:*	☐	☐	☐	
31. Record removal of disk on MAR. *Comments:*	☐	☐	☐	
Ear Medication 1. Check for allergies. *Comments:*	☐	☐	☐	
2. Check MAR against prescribing practitioner's written orders. *Comments:*	☐	☐	☐	
3. Wash hands/hand hygiene. *Comments:*	☐	☐	☐	
4. Calculate dose. *Comments:*	☐	☐	☐	

continued on the following page

continued from the previous page

Procedure 30-9 Medication Administration: Eye and Ear	Able to Perform	Able to Perform with Assistance	Unable to Perform	Initials/Date
5. Identify client by checking client's armband. *Comments:*	☐	☐	☐	
6. Explain procedure to client. *Comments:*	☐	☐	☐	
7. Place client in a side-lying position with affected ear facing up. *Comments:*	☐	☐	☐	
8. Straighten ear canal. *Comments:*	☐	☐	☐	
9. Slowly instill drops into ear canal by holding dropper at least 1/2 inch above ear canal. *Comments:*	☐	☐	☐	
10. Ask client to maintain position for 2–3 minutes. *Comments:*	☐	☐	☐	
11. Place a cotton ball on outermost part of canal. *Comments:*	☐	☐	☐	
12. Wash hands/hand hygiene. *Comments:*	☐	☐	☐	
13. Document drug, number of drops, time administered, and ear medicated. *Comments:*	☐	☐	☐	

Checklist for Procedure 30-10   Medication Administration: Nasal

Name _____   Date _____

School _____

Instructor _____

Course _____

Procedure 30-10 Medication Administration: Nasal	Able to Perform	Able to Perform with Assistance	Unable to Perform	Initials/Date
1. Wash hands/hand hygiene. Wear a mask, if needed. Put on latex-free gloves. *Comments:*	☐	☐	☐	
2. Explain procedure to client. *Comments:*	☐	☐	☐	
3. Explain to client the sensation of medication effects. *Comments:*	☐	☐	☐	
4. Explain manufacturer's directions for inhaler use. Follow five rights of drug administration. *Comments:*	☐	☐	☐	
5. Have client assume a comfortable position. Have client blow nose. Squeeze nose drops into dropper. *Comments:*	☐	☐	☐	
6. Have client exhale and close one nostril. *Comments:*	☐	☐	☐	

continued on the following page

continued from the previous page

Procedure 30-10 Medication Administration: Nasal	Able to Perform	Able to Perform with Assistance	Unable to Perform	Initials/Date
7. Ask client to inhale while spray is pumped or sprayed into first nostril. If nose drops are used, insert nasal dropper only about 3/8 inch into nostril, keeping tip of dropper away from sides of nostril. Insert prescribed dosage of medication into nostril. Discard any unused medication in dropper. *Comments:*	☐	☐	☐	
8. Ask client to blot excess drainage from nostril; do not have client blow nose. *Comments:*	☐	☐	☐	
9. Repeat procedure on other nostril. *Comments:*	☐	☐	☐	
10. Help client resume comfortable position. For nose drops, client stays in position generally 5 minutes. Instruct client to breathe through nose. *Comments:*	☐	☐	☐	
11. Remove all soiled supplies and dispose according to Standard Precautions. Remove gloves. Wash hands/hand hygiene. *Comments:*	☐	☐	☐	
12. Evaluate effect of medication in 15–20 minutes. *Comments:*	☐	☐	☐	

Checklist for Procedure 30-11 Medication Administration: Nebulizer

Name _____ Date _____

School _____

Instructor _____

Course _____

Procedure 30-11 Medication Administration: Nebulizer	Able to Perform	Able to Perform with Assistance	Unable to Perform	Initials/Date
Handheld Nebulizer 1. Assess client's ability to use nebulizer. *Comments:*	☐	☐	☐	
2. Check MAR against prescribing practitioner's orders. *Comments:*	☐	☐	☐	
3. Check for drug allergies and hypersensitivity. *Comments:*	☐	☐	☐	
4. Wash hands/hand hygiene before setting up nebulizer. Gather equipment. *Comments:*	☐	☐	☐	
5. Set up medication for one client at a time. *Comments:*	☐	☐	☐	
6. Look at medication at eye level if using droppers to dispense solution into nebulizer. *Comments:*	☐	☐	☐	
7. Pour entire amount of drug(s) into nebulizer cup carefully. • Avoid touching drug while pouring into nebulizer cup. *Comments:*	☐	☐	☐	

continued on the following page

continued from the previous page

Procedure 30-11 Medication Administration: Nebulizer	Able to Perform	Able to Perform with Assistance	Unable to Perform	Initials/Date
8. Cover cup with cap and fasten. *Comments:*	☐	☐	☐	
9. Fasten T-piece to cap top. *Comments:*	☐	☐	☐	
10. Fasten short length of tubing to one end of T-piece. *Comments:*	☐	☐	☐	
11. Fasten mouthpiece or mask to other end of T-piece. • Avoid touching nebulizer mouthpiece or interior part of mask. *Comments:*	☐	☐	☐	
12. Identify client. *Comments:*	☐	☐	☐	
13. Identify medication to client and explain its purpose. *Comments:*	☐	☐	☐	
14. Assist client to upright position. *Comments:*	☐	☐	☐	
15. Attach tubing to nebulizer cup bottom and attach other end to air source: • Adjust wall oxygen valve per prescribing practitioner's orders. • Leave air on for about 6–7 minutes until medications are used up. *Comments:*	☐	☐	☐	

continued on the following page

continued from the previous page

Procedure 30-11 Medication Administration: Nebulizer	Able to Perform	Able to Perform with Assistance	Unable to Perform	Initials/Date
16. Instruct client to breathe in and out slowly and deeply through mouthpiece or mask. • Client's lips should be sealed tightly around mouthpiece. *Comments:*	☐	☐	☐	
17. Remain with client long enough to observe proper inhalation-exhalation technique. *Comments:*	☐	☐	☐	
18. Wash hands/hand hygiene. *Comments:*	☐	☐	☐	
19. Record medications administered with date, time, and dosages on chart. *Comments:*	☐	☐	☐	
20. When nebulizer cup empty, turn off compressor or wall air. • Detach tubing from compressor and nebulizer. • If nebulizer disposable, dispose of it in appropriate container. • If nebulizer to be reused for this client, carefully wash, rinse, and dry nebulizer components. *Comments:*	☐	☐	☐	
21. Assess client immediately following treatment for results or adverse effects from treatment. *Comments:*	☐	☐	☐	
22. Reassess client 5–10 minutes following treatment. *Comments:*	☐	☐	☐	

continued on the following page

continued from the previous page

Procedure 30-11 Medication Administration: Nebulizer	Able to Perform	Able to Perform with Assistance	Unable to Perform	Initials/Date
23. Wash hands/hand hygiene. *Comments:*	☐	☐	☐	
Metered-Dose Nebulizer 24. Assess client for ability to use metered-dose nebulizer. *Comments:*	☐	☐	☐	
25. Check medication administration record against prescribing practitioner's orders. *Comments:*	☐	☐	☐	
26. Check for drug allergies and hypersensitivity. *Comments:*	☐	☐	☐	
27. Wash hands/hand hygiene before administering medication; put on latex-free gloves. *Comments:*	☐	☐	☐	
28. Shake prepackaged nebulizer. *Comments:*	☐	☐	☐	
29. Place nebulizer into applicator. *Comments:*	☐	☐	☐	
30. Place aerochamber onto nebulizer, if needed. *Comments:*	☐	☐	☐	
31. Have client place mouthpiece in mouth. *Comments:*	☐	☐	☐	

continued on the following page

continued from the previous page

Procedure 30-11 Medication Administration: Nebulizer	Able to Perform	Able to Perform with Assistance	Unable to Perform	Initials/Date
32. Have client press down on prepackaged dispenser as client simultaneously inhales. *Comments:*	☐	☐	☐	
33. If an aerochamber is attached to nebulizer, have client inhale slowly and deeply. *Comments:*	☐	☐	☐	
34. Observe client for possible adverse effects. *Comments:*	☐	☐	☐	
35. Wash hands/hand hygiene. *Comments:*	☐	☐	☐	
36. Record medication administration and observations. *Comments:*	☐	☐	☐	

Checklist for Procedure 30-12   Medication Administration: Rectal

Name _____ Date _____

School _____

Instructor _____

Course _____

Procedure 30-12 Medication Administration: Rectal	Able to Perform	Able to Perform with Assistance	Unable to Perform	Initials/Date
1. Assess client's need for medication. *Comments:*	☐	☐	☐	
2. Check prescribing practitioner's written order. *Comments:*	☐	☐	☐	
3. Check MAR against medication order, verifying correct client, medication, dose, route, and time. *Comments:*	☐	☐	☐	
4. Check for drug allergies. *Comments:*	☐	☐	☐	
5. Review client's history. *Comments:*	☐	☐	☐	
6. Gather equipment. *Comments:*	☐	☐	☐	
7. Assess client's readiness. Ask visitors to leave. Provide for privacy. *Comments:*	☐	☐	☐	
8. Wash hands/hand hygiene. *Comments:*	☐	☐	☐	

continued on the following page

continued from the previous page

Procedure 30-12 Medication Administration: Rectal	Able to Perform	Able to Perform with Assistance	Unable to Perform	Initials/Date
9. Apply disposable gloves. *Comments:*	☐	☐	☐	
10. Ask client's name and check identification band. *Comments:*	☐	☐	☐	
11. Assist client into correct position; side-lying Sims' position. Place towel or pad under client. *Comments:*	☐	☐	☐	
12. Visually assess client's external anus. *Comments:*	☐	☐	☐	
13. Remove suppository from wrapper and lubricate rounded end along with insertion finger. If a medicated enema is used, lubricate enema tip, if needed. *Comments:*	☐	☐	☐	
14. Tell client to expect a cool sensation and pressure during administration. Encourage slow deep breaths. *Comments:*	☐	☐	☐	
15. Retract buttocks with nondominant hand, visualizing anus. Using dominant index finger, slowly and gently insert suppository through anus, past internal sphincter, and against rectal wall. Depth of insertion will differ if client is a child or infant. If instilling a medicated enema, gently insert enema tip past internal sphincter and instill the contents by slowly squeezing. *Comments:*	☐	☐	☐	

continued on the following page

continued from the previous page

Procedure 30-12 Medication Administration: Rectal	Able to Perform	Able to Perform with Assistance	Unable to Perform	Initials/Date
16. Remove finger or enema tip and wipe client's anal area with a washcloth or tissue. *Comments:*	☐	☐	☐	
17. Discard gloves. *Comments:*	☐	☐	☐	
18. Discuss with client a 10-minute time frame to remain in bed or on side. *Comments:*	☐	☐	☐	
19. Place call light in client's reach. *Comments:*	☐	☐	☐	
20. Record administration of medication. *Comments:*	☐	☐	☐	
21. Document treatment results. *Comments:*	☐	☐	☐	
22. Wash hands/hand hygiene. *Comments:*	☐	☐	☐	

Checklist for Procedure 30-13 Medication Administration: Vaginal

Name _____ Date _____

School _____

Instructor _____

Course _____

Procedure 30-13 Medication Administration: Vaginal	Able to Perform	Able to Perform with Assistance	Unable to Perform	Initials/Date
1. Verify orders. Comments:	☐	☐	☐	
2. Assess client's level of knowledge of procedure. Comments:	☐	☐	☐	
3. Ask client to void. Comments:	☐	☐	☐	
4. Wash hands/hand hygiene. Comments:	☐	☐	☐	
5. Gather equipment and arrange at client's bedside. Comments:	☐	☐	☐	
6. Provide privacy. Comments:	☐	☐	☐	
7. Assist client to a dorsal-recumbent or Sims' position. Comments:	☐	☐	☐	
8. Drape client as appropriate, Provide towel or protective pad on bed. Comments:	☐	☐	☐	

continued on the following page

continued from the previous page

Procedure 30-13 Medication Administration: Vaginal	Able to Perform	Able to Perform with Assistance	Unable to Perform	Initials/Date
9. Position lighting to illuminate vaginal orifice. *Comments:*	☐	☐	☐	
10. Put on latex-free gloves and assess perineal area for redness, inflammation, discharge, or foul odor. *Comments:*	☐	☐	☐	
11. If using an applicator, fill with medication. If using a suppository, remove suppository from foil and position in applicator (applicator is optional). Discard foil. Apply water-soluble lubricant to suppository or applicator (optional for applicator). *Comments:*	☐	☐	☐	
12. For suppository, with nondominant hand, retract labia. *Comments:*	☐	☐	☐	
13. With dominant hand, insert applicator 2–3 inches into vagina, sliding applicator posteriorly. Push plunger to administer medication. With a suppository, insert tapered end first with index finger or applicator along posterior wall of vagina (approximately 3 inches). *Comments:*	☐	☐	☐	
14. Withdraw applicator and place on towel. *Comments:*	☐	☐	☐	

continued on the following page

continued from the previous page

Procedure 30-13 Medication Administration: Vaginal	Able to Perform	Able to Perform with Assistance	Unable to Perform	Initials/Date
15. If administering douche or irrigation: • Warm solution to slightly above body temperature. Check using back of hand or wrist. • Position client in semirecumbent position on bedpan, toilet seat, or in tub. • Apply lubricant to irrigation nozzle and insert approximately 3 inches into vagina. • Hang irrigant container approximately 2 feet above client's vaginal area. • Open clamp and allow small amount of solution to flow into vagina. • Move nozzle and rotate around entire vaginal area. If labia are inflamed, allow solution to flow over labia as well. If client is on toilet seat, alternate between closing off labia and allowing solution to be expelled. *Comments:*	☐	☐	☐	
16. Wipe and clean client's perineal area, including labia (from front to back) with toilet tissue or warm cloth and water. *Comments:*	☐	☐	☐	
17. Apply a perineal pad. *Comments:*	☐	☐	☐	
18. Wash applicator (if reusable) with soap and warm water and store in appropriate container in client's room. *Comments:*	☐	☐	☐	
19. Remove gloves; wash hands/hand hygiene. *Comments:*	☐	☐	☐	

continued on the following page

continued from the previous page

Procedure 30-13 Medication Administration: Vaginal	Able to Perform	Able to Perform with Assistance	Unable to Perform	Initials/Date
20. Instruct client to remain flat for at least 30 minutes. *Comments:*	☐	☐	☐	
21. Raise side rails and place call light in reach. *Comments:*	☐	☐	☐	
22. Wash hands/hand hygiene. *Comments:*	☐	☐	☐	

Checklist for Procedure 31-1   Administering Therapeutic Massage

Name _____ Date _____

School _____

Instructor _____

Course _____

Procedure 31-1 Administering Therapeutic Massage	Able to Perform	Able to Perform with Assistance	Unable to Perform	Initials/Date
1. Set room temperature at 75°F. Provide low lighting, privacy, and background music. *Comments:*	☐	☐	☐	
2. Prepare table or hospital bed. *Comments:*	☐	☐	☐	
3. Remove rings and watch. Wash hands. *Comments:*	☐	☐	☐	
4. Explain procedure to client. *Comments:*	☐	☐	☐	
5. Assist client to assume either a prone, Sim's, or sitting position, depending on client's condition. *Comments:*	☐	☐	☐	
6. Loosen or remove clothing from client's back and arms. Drape client with sheet, as needed. *Comments:*				
7. Squeeze small amount of lotion or oil into palm of hand to warm. *Comments:*	☐	☐	☐	

continued on the following page

continued from the previous page

Procedure 31-1 Administering Therapeutic Massage	Able to Perform	Able to Perform with Assistance	Unable to Perform	Initials/Date
8. Begin with light to medium effleurage at lower back and continue upward following muscle groups, being careful to avoid spine and spinal processes. Move hands up toward base of neck and continue outward over trapezius muscles with circular motions, over and around shoulders and upper arms, and return with lighter downward strokes laterally over latissimus dorsi to upper gluteals. Use slow rhythmic movements, keeping in contact with skin at all times. Check pressure. Continue effleurage for approximately 3 minutes. *Comments:*	☐	☐	☐	
9. Continue treatment, if appropriate, with gentle petrissage to major muscle groups in back, shoulders, and upper arms. *Comments:*	☐	☐	☐	
10. Use friction to particular muscle groups where tension is being held. *Comments:*	☐	☐	☐	
11. Use tapotement to stimulate any fatigued muscle groups. *Comments:*	☐	☐	☐	
12. Finish treatment with effleurage. *Comments:*	☐	☐	☐	
13. Wipe any excess lotion or oil from skin or use warm soap and water to clean client's skin, then dry completely. *Comments:*	☐	☐	☐	

continued on the following page

continued from the previous page

Procedure 31-1 Administering Therapeutic Massage	Able to Perform	Able to Perform with Assistance	Unable to Perform	Initials/Date
14. Assist client into comfortable position. *Comments:*	☐	☐	☐	
15. Document treatment, client's response, and skin assessment data. *Comments:*	☐	☐	☐	
18. Wash hands/hand hygiene. *Comments:*	☐	☐	☐	

Checklist for Procedure 32-1   Maintaining and Cleaning the Tracheostomy Tube

Name _____ Date _____

School _____

Instructor _____

Course _____

Procedure 32-1 Maintaining and Cleaning the Tracheostomy Tube	Able to Perform	Able to Perform with Assistance	Unable to Perform	Initials/Date
Cleaning Trach Tube Site 1. Hand hygiene, apply gloves, and assemble equipment. *Comments:*	☐	☐	☐	
2. Remove soiled dressing and discard. *Comments:*	☐	☐	☐	
3. Cleanse neck plate of tracheostomy tube with cotton applicators moistened with hydrogen peroxide. *Comments*	☐	☐	☐	
4. Rinse neck plate of tracheostomy tube with applicators moistened with sterile water or saline. *Comments:*	☐	☐	☐	
5. Cleanse skin under neck plate of tube with cotton applicator moistened with hydrogen peroxide. *Comments:*	☐	☐	☐	
6. Rinse skin under neck plate with applicators moistened with sterile water or saline. *Comments:*	☐	☐	☐	
7. Dry skin under neck plate with cotton applicators. *Comments:*	☐	☐	☐	

continued on the following page

continued from the previous page

Procedure 32-1 Maintaining and Cleaning the Tracheostomy Tube	Able to Perform	Able to Perform with Assistance	Unable to Perform	Initials/Date
8. *Using your clean hand*, gently loosen inner cannula of tracheostomy tube by twisting outer ring counterclockwise; then withdraw inner cannula in smooth motion. Place inner cannula into basin of peroxide. *Comments:*	☐	☐	☐	
9. Using your sterile hand, pick up cannula. Using your clean hand, pick up nylon brush and scrub to remove any visible crusts or secretions from inside and outside cannula. *Comments:*	☐	☐	☐	
10. Place cannula into container of sterile saline. Agitate so all surfaces are bathed in saline. *Comments:*	☐	☐	☐	
11. Inspect inner cannula again to ensure is clean; then remove excess saline from lumen by tapping cannula against a sterile surface. *Comments:*	☐	☐	☐	
12. Gently replace inner cannula, following curve of tube. When fully inserted, lock inner cannula in place by rotating external ring clockwise until clicks into place. *Comments:*	☐	☐	☐	
13. Prepare clean tracheostomy ties. • Cut length of twill tape that will fit around client's neck plus 6 inches. Cut ends of twill tape on diagonal.	☐	☐	☐	

continued on the following page

continued from the previous page

Procedure 32-1 Maintaining and Cleaning the Tracheostomy Tube	Able to Perform	Able to Perform with Assistance	Unable to Perform	Initials/Date
• Open Velcro ties on continuous neckband. *Comments:*				
14. Leaving old tracheostomy ties in place, insert one end of new tracheostomy tie through hole in tracheostomy neck plate from back to front. Pull ends even, and slid ends of tape around back to other side. *Comments:*	☐	☐	☐	
15. Insert one end of tape through opening on other side of tracheostomy tube neck plate from back to front. *Comments:*	☐	☐	☐	
16. Tie two ends of new tape with a square knot. Keep two fingers under tape as the knot is tied. Without putting pressure on neck plate or the tape, pull on knot to make sure it will stay tied. *Comments:*	☐	☐	☐	
17. Untie and remove old tracheostomy tapes and discard. Hold neck plate firmly with one hand while untying old tapes. *Comments:*	☐	☐	☐	
18. Place one finger under tracheostomy ties. *Comments:*	☐	☐	☐	

continued on the following page

continued from the previous page

Procedure 32-1 **Maintaining and Cleaning the Tracheostomy Tube**	**Able to Perform**	**Able to Perform with Assistance**	**Unable to Perform**	**Initials/Date**
Two-Person Technique of Changing Tracheostomy Ties 19. Cut two pieces of twill tape about 12 to 14 inches in length. *Comments:*	☐	☐	☐	
20. Make fold 1 inch below end of each piece of twill tape and cut 1/2- inch slit lengthwise in center of fold. *Comments:*	☐	☐	☐	
21. Have second person hold tracheostomy tube with fingers on sides of neck plate. *Comments:*	☐	☐	☐	
22. Untie old tracheostomy ties and discard. *Comments:*	☐	☐	☐	
23. Insert split end of tracheostomy tape through opening on one side of tracheostomy tube neck plate. Pull distal end of tracheostomy tie through cut end and pull tightly. *Comments:*	☐	☐	☐	
24. Repeat procedure with second piece of twill tape. *Comments:*	☐	☐	☐	
25. Tie tracheostomy tapes with a double knot at side of neck. *Comments:*	☐	☐	☐	
26. Insert one finger under tracheostomy tapes. *Comments:*	☐	☐	☐	

continued on the following page

continued from the previous page

Procedure 32-1 Maintaining and Cleaning the Tracheostomy Tube	Able to Perform	Able to Perform with Assistance	Unable to Perform	Initials/Date
27. Insert tracheostomy gauze under neck plate of tube. *Comments:*	☐	☐	☐	
28. Discard all used materials and hand hygiene. *Comments:*	☐	☐	☐	

Checklist for Procedure 32-2   Performing Nasopharyngeal and Oropharyngeal Suctioning

Name _____ Date _____

School _____

Instructor _____

Course _____

Procedure 32-2 Performing Nasopharyngeal and Oropharyngeal Suctioning	Able to Perform	Able to Perform with Assistance	Unable to Perform	Initials/Date
1. Assess client's need for suctioning: inability to clear airway by coughing and expectoration; coarse bubbling or gurgling noises with respiration. *Comments:*	☐	☐	☐	
2. Choose appropriate route. If nasopharyngeal approach, inspect nares with penlight to determine patency. Assess patency by occluding each nare, in turn, with finger pressure while asking client to breathe through other nare. *Comments:*	☐	☐	☐	
3. Explain procedure to client. Advise suctioning can cause coughing or gagging but emphasize importance of clearing airway. *Comments:*	☐	☐	☐	
4. Wash hands/hand hygiene. *Comments:*	☐	☐	☐	
5. Position client in a high Fowler's or semi-Fowler's position. *Comments:*	☐	☐	☐	
6. If client unconscious or otherwise unable to protect airway, place in a side-lying position. *Comments:*	☐	☐	☐	

continued on the following page

continued from the previous page

Procedure 32-2 **Performing Nasopharyngeal and Oropharyngeal Suctioning**	**Able to Perform**	**Able to Perform with Assistance**	**Unable to Perform**	**Initials/Date**
7. Connect extension tubing to suction device and adjust suction control to between 80 and 100 mm Hg. *Comments:*	☐	☐	☐	
8. Put on gown, mask, and goggles or face shield, if indicated. *Comments:*	☐	☐	☐	
9. Using sterile technique, open suction kit. Consider inside wrapper of kit sterile, and spread wrapper out to create a small sterile field. *Comments:*	☐	☐	☐	
10. Open packet of sterile water-soluble lubricant and squeeze out contents of packet onto sterile field. *Comments:*	☐	☐	☐	
11. If sterile solution (water or saline) is included in kit, pour about 100 ml of solution into sterile container provided in kit. *Comments:*	☐	☐	☐	
12. Carefully lift wrapped gloves from kit without touching inside of kit or gloves. Lay wrapped gloves next to suction kit and open wrapper. Put on gloves using sterile gloving technique. *Comments:*	☐	☐	☐	
13. Open cup of sterile solution, if included in suction kit. *Comments:*	☐	☐	☐	

continued on the following page

continued from the previous page

Procedure 32-2 Performing Nasopharyngeal and Oropharyngeal Suctioning	Able to Perform	Able to Perform with Assistance	Unable to Perform	Initials/Date
14. Designate one hand as sterile and other as clean. *Comments:*	☐	☐	☐	
15. Using sterile hand, pick up suction catheter. Grasp plastic connector end between thumb and forefinger and coil tip around remaining fingers. *Comments:*	☐	☐	☐	
16. Pick up extension tubing with clean hand. Connect suction catheter to extension tubing, taking care not to contaminate catheter. *Comments:*	☐	☐	☐	
17. Position clean hand with thumb over catheter's suction port. *Comments:*	☐	☐	☐	
18. Dip catheter tip into sterile solution, and activate suction. Observe as solution is drawn into catheter. *Comments:*	☐	☐	☐	
19. For oropharyngeal suctioning, ask client to open mouth. Without activating suction, gently insert catheter and advance until pool of secretions is reached or until client coughs. *Comments:*	☐	☐	☐	
20. For nasopharyngeal suctioning, estimate distance from tip of client's nose to earlobe and grasp catheter between thumb and forefinger at a point equal to this distance from catheter's tip. *Comments:*	☐	☐	☐	

continued on the following page

continued from the previous page

Procedure 32-2 Performing Nasopharyngeal and Oropharyngeal Suctioning	Able to Perform	Able to Perform with Assistance	Unable to Perform	Initials/Date
21. Dip tip of suction catheter into water-soluble lubricant. *Comments:*	☐	☐	☐	
22. Insert catheter tip into nare with suction control port uncovered. Advance catheter gently with slight downward slant. Slight rotation of catheter may ease insertion. Advance catheter to point marked by thumb and forefinger. *Comments:*	☐	☐	☐	
23. If resistance is met, *do not force catheter.* Withdraw and attempt insertion via opposite nare. *Comments:*	☐	☐	☐	
24. Apply suction intermittently by occluding suction control port with thumb; at same time, slowly rotate catheter by rolling between thumb and fingers while slowly withdrawing. Apply suction for no longer than 15 seconds at a time. *Comments:*	☐	☐	☐	
25. Repeat Action 24 until secretions are cleared, allowing brief rest periods between suctioning episodes. *Comments:*	☐	☐	☐	
26. Withdraw catheter by looping around fingers as removed. *Comments:*	☐	☐	☐	
27. Dip catheter tip into sterile solution and apply suction. *Comments:*	☐	☐	☐	

continued on the following page

continued from the previous page

Procedure 32-2 **Performing Nasopharyngeal and Oropharyngeal Suctioning**	**Able to Perform**	**Able to Perform with Assistance**	**Unable to Perform**	**Initials/Date**
28. Disconnect catheter from extension tubing. Holding coiled catheter in gloved hand, remove glove by pulling over catheter. Discard catheter and gloves in appropriate container. *Comments:*	☐	☐	☐	
29. Discard remaining supplies in appropriate container. *Comments:*	☐	☐	☐	
30. Wash hands/hand hygiene. *Comments:*	☐	☐	☐	
31. Provide client with oral hygiene, if needed or desired. *Comments:*	☐	☐	☐	
32. Document procedure, noting amount, color, and odor of secretions and client's response to procedure. *Comments:*	☐	☐	☐	

Checklist for Procedure 32-3   Suctioning Endotracheal and Tracheal Tubes

Name _____ Date _____

School _____

Instructor _____

Course _____

Procedure 32-3 Suctioning Endotracheal and Tracheal Tubes	Able to Perform	Able to Perform with Assistance	Unable to Perform	Initials/Date
Suctioning a Tracheal Tube				
1. Assess depth and rate of respirations; auscultate breath sounds. *Comments:*	☐	☐	☐	
2. Assemble supplies. *Comments:*	☐	☐	☐	
3. Wash hands/hand hygiene. *Comments:*	☐	☐	☐	
4. Connect suction tube to source of negative pressure. Set suction control between 80 and 100 mm Hg. *Comments:*	☐	☐	☐	
5. Administer oxygen or use Ambubag before beginning procedure. *Comments:*	☐	☐	☐	
6. Remove inner cannula and place in basin of hydrogen peroxide to loosen secretions, if reusable, or set aside if disposable. Do not dispose of disposable cannula until new inner cannula is securely in place. *Comments:*	☐	☐	☐	
7. Apply sterile glove to dominant hand. *Comments:*	☐	☐	☐	

continued on the following page

continued from the previous page

Procedure 32-3 Suctioning Endotracheal and Tracheal Tubes	Able to Perform	Able to Perform with Assistance	Unable to Perform	Initials/Date
8. Open sterile suction catheter or use reusable closed system catheter. Remove sterile suction catheter from package with dominant, sterile hand. Wrap catheter tubing around hand from tip of catheter down to port end. Attach catheter to suction. *Comments:*	☐	☐	☐	
9. Insert catheter into trachea without suction. *Comments:*	☐	☐	☐	
10. Apply suction intermittently while gently rotating catheter and removing it. • In a disposable catheter, suction is applied by placing thumb of dominant hand over open port of catheter connector. • In a closed system catheter, suction is applied by depressing white button at connector end of catheter. *Comments:*	☐	☐	☐	
11. Wrap disposable suction catheter around sterile dominant hand while withdrawing from the endotracheal tube. *Comments:*	☐	☐	☐	
12. Suction for no more than 10 seconds. *Comments:*	☐	☐	☐	
13. Administer oxygen using the sigh function on ventilator or an Ambubag. *Comments:*	☐	☐	☐	

continued on the following page

continued from the previous page

Procedure 32-3 Suctioning Endotracheal and Tracheal Tubes	Able to Perform	Able to Perform with Assistance	Unable to Perform	Initials/Date
14. Assess airway and repeat suctioning, as necessary. *Comments:*	☐	☐	☐	
15. Clean inner cannula using tracheostomy brush and rinse well in sterile water or sterile saline. Dry (or open new disposable inner cannula). *Comments:*	☐	☐	☐	
16. Reinsert inner cannula and lock into place. *Comments:*	☐	☐	☐	
17. Apply humidified oxygen or compressed air. *Comments:*	☐	☐	☐	
18. Remove gloves and discard. *Comments:*	☐	☐	☐	
19. Wash hands/hand hygiene. *Comments:*	☐	☐	☐	
20. Record procedure and client's tolerance of procedure, including amount and consistency of secretions. *Comments:*	☐	☐	☐	
Suctioning an Endotracheal Tube 21. Repeat Actions 1–14. *Comments:*	☐	☐	☐	
22. Remove gloves and discard. *Comments:*	☐	☐	☐	

continued on the following page

continued from the previous page

Procedure 32-3 Suctioning Endotracheal and Tracheal Tubes	Able to Perform	Able to Perform with Assistance	Unable to Perform	Initials/Date
23. Wash hands/hand hygiene. *Comments:*	☐	☐	☐	
24. Record procedure and client's tolerance of procedure, including amount and consistency of secretions. *Comments:*	☐	☐	☐	

continued on the following page

Checklist for Procedure 32-4   Administering Oxygen Therapy

Name _____ Date _____

School _____

Instructor _____

Course _____

Procedure 32-4 Administering Oxygen Therapy	Able to Perform	Able to Perform with Assistance	Unable to Perform	Initials/Date
Nasal Cannula 1. Wash hands/hand hygiene. *Comments:*	☐	☐	☐	
2. Verify prescribing practitioner's order. *Comments:*	☐	☐	☐	
3. Explain procedure and hazards to client. Remind clients who smoke of reasons for not smoking while O_2 is in use. *Comments:*	☐	☐	☐	
4. If using humidity, fill humidifier to fill line with distilled water and close container. *Comments:*	☐	☐	☐	
5. Attach humidifier to oxygen flow meter. *Comments:*	☐	☐	☐	
6. Insert humidifier and flow meter into oxygen source in wall or portable unit. *Comments:*	☐	☐	☐	
7. Attach oxygen tubing and nasal cannula to flow meter and turn it on to tprescribed flow rate. Use extension tubing for ambulatory clients. *Comments:*	☐	☐	☐	

continued on the following page

continued from the previous page

Procedure 32-4 Administering Oxygen Therapy	Able to Perform	Able to Perform with Assistance	Unable to Perform	Initials/Date
8. Check for bubbling in humidifier. *Comments:*	☐	☐	☐	
9. Place nasal prongs in client's nostrils. Secure cannula in place by adjusting tubing around client's ears and using slip ring to stabilize under client's chin. *Comments:*	☐	☐	☐	
10. Check for proper flow rate every 4 hours and when client returns from procedures. *Comments:*	☐	☐	☐	
11. Assess client's nostrils every 8 hours. If client complains of dryness or has signs of irritation, use sterile lubricant to keep mucous membranes moist. Add humidifier, if not already in place. *Comments:*	☐	☐	☐	
12. Monitor vital signs, oxygen saturation, and client's condition every 4–8 hours (or as indicated or ordered) for signs and symptoms of hypoxia. *Comments:*	☐	☐	☐	
13. Wean client from oxygen as soon as possible, using standard protocols. *Comments:*	☐	☐	☐	
Mask: Venturi (High Flow Device), Simple Mask (Low Flow), Partial Rebreather Mask, Nonrebreather Mask, and Face Tent 14. Wash hands/hand hygiene. *Comments:*	☐	☐	☐	

continued on the following page

continued from the previous page

Procedure 32-4 Administering Oxygen Therapy	Able to Perform	Able to Perform with Assistance	Unable to Perform	Initials/Date
15. Repeat Actions 2–6. Comments:	☐	☐	☐	
16. Attach appropriately sized mask or face tent to oxygen tubing and turn on flow meter to prescribed flow rate. Allow reservoir bag of nonrebreathing or partial rebreathing mask to fill completely. Comments:	☐	☐	☐	
17. Check for bubbling in humidifier. Comments:	☐	☐	☐	
18. Place mask or tent on client's face; fasten elastic band around client's ears and tighten until mask fits snugly. Comments:	☐	☐	☐	
19. Check for proper flow rate every 4 hours. Comments:	☐	☐	☐	
20. Ensure that ports of Venturi mask are not under covers or impeded by any other source. Comments:	☐	☐	☐	
21. Assess client's face and ears for pressure from mask and use padding, as needed. Comments:	☐	☐	☐	
22. Wean client to nasal cannula and then wean off oxygen per protocol. Comments:	☐	☐	☐	

continued on the following page

continued from the previous page

Procedure 32-4 Administering Oxygen Therapy	Able to Perform	Able to Perform with Assistance	Unable to Perform	Initials/Date
Oxygen Via an Artificial Airway (Tracheostomy or Endotracheal Tube) 23. Wash hands/hand hygiene. *Comments:*	☐	☐	☐	
24. Verify the prescribing practitioner's order. *Comments:*	☐	☐	☐	
25. Fill humidifier with sterile water and close container. *Comments:*	☐	☐	☐	
26. Attach humidifier and warmer to oxygen flow meter. *Comments:*	☐	☐	☐	
27. Attach wide bore oxygen tubing and T-tube adapter or tracheostomy mask to flow meter and turn meter to flow rate needed to achieve prescribed oxygen concentration. *Comments:*	☐	☐	☐	
28. Check for bubbling in humidifier and fine mist from the adapter. *Comments:*	☐	☐	☐	
29. Attach T-piece to client's artificial airway or place mask over client's airway. Be sure T-piece is firmly attached to airway. *Comments:*	☐	☐	☐	

continued on the following page

continued from the previous page

Procedure 32-4 Administering Oxygen Therapy	Able to Perform	Able to Perform with Assistance	Unable to Perform	Initials/Date
30. Position tubing so that it is not pulling client's airway. *Comments:*	☐	☐	☐	
31. Check for proper flow rate and patency of system every 1–2 hours, depending on client acuity. Suction as needed. *Comments:*	☐	☐	☐	
32. Monitor airway patency, vital signs, oxygen saturation, and for signs and symptoms of hypoxia every 2 hours, or as needed. Additionally, monitor breath sounds and tube position every 4 hours. *Comments:*	☐	☐	☐	
33. Wean client from therapy as directed by prescribing practitioner. *Comments:*	☐	☐	☐	

Checklist for Procedure 32-5   Performing the Heimlich Maneuver

Name _____ Date _____

School _____

Instructor _____

Course _____

Procedure 32-5 Performing the Heimlich Maneuver	Able to Perform	Able to Perform with Assistance	Unable to Perform	Initials/Date
Foreign Body Obstruction—All Clients 1. Assess airway for complete or partial blockage. *Comments:*	☐	☐	☐	
2. Activate emergency response assistance if respiratory distress or complete blockage; for example, ask bystander to call 911. *Comments:*	☐	☐	☐	
Conscious Adult Client—Sitting or Standing (Heimlich Maneuver) 3. Stand behind client. *Comments:*	☐	☐	☐	
4. Wrap both arms around client's waist. *Comments:*	☐	☐	☐	
5. Make fist with one hand and grasp fist with other hand, placing thumb side of fist against client's abdomen. Place fist midline, below xiphoid process and lower margins of rib cage, above navel. *Comments:*	☐	☐	☐	
6. Perform a quick upward thrust into client's abdomen. *Comments:*	☐	☐	☐	

continued on the following page

continued from the previous page

Procedure 32-5 Performing the Heimlich Maneuver	Able to Perform	Able to Perform with Assistance	Unable to Perform	Initials/Date
7. Repeat process 6–10 times until client either expels foreign body or loses consciousness. *Comments:*	☐	☐	☐	
Unconscious Adult Client or Adult Client Who Becomes Unconscious 8. Repeat Actions 1 and 2. *Comments:*	☐	☐	☐	
9. Position client supine; kneel astride client's abdomen. *Comments:*	☐	☐	☐	
10. Place heel of one hand midline, below xiphoid process and lower margin of rib cage, above navel. Place second hand directly on top of first hand. *Comments:*	☐	☐	☐	
11. Perform quick upward thrust into diaphragm, repeating 6–10 times. *Comments:*	☐	☐	☐	
12. Perform a finger sweep: a. Use one hand to grasp lower jaw and tongue between thumb and fingers and lift. b. Using index finger of other hand, insert finger into client's mouth next to cheek and, using a hooking motion, dislodge any foreign body. Use caution to prevent pushing foreign body farther down into airway. *Comments:*	☐	☐	☐	

continued on the following page

continued from the previous page

Procedure 32-5 **Performing the Heimlich Maneuver**	Able to Perform	Able to Perform with Assistance	Unable to Perform	Initials/Date
13. Open client's airway and attempt ventilation. *Comments:*	☐	☐	☐	
14. Continue sequence of Heimlich maneuver, finger sweep, and rescue breathing as long as necessary. *Comments:*	☐	☐	☐	
Conscious Adult Sitting or Standing— Chest Thrusts 15. Repeat Actions 1 and 2. *Comments:*	☐	☐	☐	
16. Stand behind client and wrap arms around client's waist. *Comments:*	☐	☐	☐	
17. Make a fist and place thumb side of fist against client's abdomen. Grasp fist with other hand upward. *Comments:*	☐	☐	☐	
18. Perform backward thrusts until client either becomes unconscious or foreign body is expelled. *Comments:*	☐	☐	☐	
Unconscious Adult—Chest Thrusts 19. Repeat Actions 1 and 2. *Comments:*	☐	☐	☐	
20. Place client in supine position and kneel astride client's thighs. *Comments:*	☐	☐	☐	

continued on the following page

continued from the previous page

Procedure 32-5 Performing the Heimlich Maneuver	Able to Perform	Able to Perform with Assistance	Unable to Perform	Initials/Date
21. Place heel of one hand against client's abdomen, slightly above navel, but below xiphoid process. *Comments:*	☐	☐	☐	
22. Perform each thrust in slow, separate, and distinct manner. *Comments:*	☐	☐	☐	
23. Follow Actions 9–12 for adult Heimlich maneuver, unconscious client. *Comments:*	☐	☐	☐	
Airway Obstruction—Infants and Small Children 24. Differentiate between infection and airway obstruction. *Comments:*	☐	☐	☐	
Infant Airway Obstruction 25. Straddle infant over forearm in prone position with head lower than trunk. Support infant's head, positioning a hand around jaws and chest. *Comments:*	☐	☐	☐	
26. Deliver 5 back blows between infant's shoulder blades. *Comments:*	☐	☐	☐	
27. Keeping infant's head down, place free hand on infant's back and turn infant over, supporting infant's back with hand and thigh. *Comments:*	☐	☐	☐	

continued on the following page

continued from the previous page

Procedure 32-5 **Performing the Heimlich Maneuver**	**Able to Perform**	**Able to Perform with Assistance**	**Unable to Perform**	**Initials/Date**
28. With free hand, deliver 5 thrusts in same manner as infant external cardiac compressions. *Comments:*	☐	☐	☐	
29. Assess for a foreign body in mouth of an unconscious infant and utilize finger sweep only if foreign body is visualized. *Comments:*	☐	☐	☐	
30. Open airway and assess for respiration. If respirations are absent, attempt rescue breathing. Assess for rise and fall of chest; if not seen, reposition infant and attempt rescue breathing again. *Comments:*	☐	☐	☐	
31. Repeat entire sequence again: 5 back blows, 5 chest thrusts, assessment for foreign body in oral cavity, and rescue breathing as long as necessary. *Comments:*	☐	☐	☐	
Small Child Airway Obstruction (Conscious, Standing, or Sitting) 32. Assess air exchange and encourage coughing and breathing. Provide reassurance to child that you are there to help. *Comments:*	☐	☐	☐	
33. Ask child if choking. If response is yes, follow steps outlined below: a. Stand behind child with arms wrapped around waist and administer 6–10 subdiaphragmatic abdominal thrusts.	☐	☐	☐	

continued on the following page

continued from the previous page

Procedure 32-5 Performing the Heimlich Maneuver	Able to Perform	Able to Perform with Assistance	Unable to Perform	Initials/Date
b. Continue until foreign object is expelled or child becomes unconscious. *Comments:*				
Small Child Airway Obstruction (Unconscious) 34. Position child supine, kneel at child's feet, and gently deliver 5 subdiaphragmatic abdominal thrusts. *Comments:*	☐	☐	☐	
35. Open airway by lifting lower jaw and tongue forward. Perform finger sweep only if foreign body is visualized. *Comments:*	☐	☐	☐	
36. If breathing is absent, begin rescue breathing. If chest does not rise, reposition child and attempt rescue breathing again. *Comments:*	☐	☐	☐	
37. Repeat this sequence as long as necessary. *Comments:*	☐	☐	☐	
38. Wash hands/hand hygiene. *Comments:*	☐	☐	☐	

Checklist for Procedure 32-6 Administering Cardiopulmonary Resuscitation (CPR)

Name _____ Date _____

School _____

Instructor _____

Course _____

Procedure 32-6 Administering Cardiopulmonary Resuscitation (CPR)	Able to Perform	Able to Perform with Assistance	Unable to Perform	Initials/Date
CPR: One Rescuer—Adult, Adolescent 1. Assess responsiveness by tapping or gently shaking client while shouting, "Are you OK?" *Comments:*	☐	☐	☐	
2. Activate emergency medical system (EMS): • In clinical setting, follow institutional protocol. • In community or home environment, activate local emergency response system (e.g., 911). *Comments:*	☐	☐	☐	
3. Position client in a supine position on hard, flat surface. *Comments:*	☐	☐	☐	
4. Apply gloves or face shield, if available. *Comments:*	☐	☐	☐	
5. Position self. Face client on knees parallel to client, next to head, to begin to assess airway and breathing status. *Comments:*	☐	☐	☐	
6. Open airway. • If head or neck injury suspected, use jaw thrust method. *Comments:*	☐	☐	☐	

continued on the following page

continued from the previous page

Procedure 32-6 **Administering Cardiopulmonary Resuscitation (CPR)**	Able to Perform	Able to Perform with Assistance	Unable to Perform	Initials/Date
7. Assess for respirations. Look, listen, and feel for air movement (3–5 seconds). *Comments:*	☐	☐	☐	
8. If respirations are absent: • Occlude nostrils with thumb and index finger of hand on forehead that is tilting head back. • Form a seal over the client's mouth using either your mouth or the appropriate respiratory assist device (e.g., Ambu(r)-bag and mask) and give two full breaths of approximately 0.5–2 seconds, allowing time for both inspiration and expiration. • In serious mouth or jaw injury that prevents mouth-to-mouth ventilation, use mouth-to-nose ventilation. *Comments:*	☐	☐	☐	
9. Assess for rise and fall of chest: • If chest rises and falls, continue to Action 10. • If chest does not move, assess for excessive oral secretions, vomit, airway obstruction, or improper positioning. *Comments:*	☐	☐	☐	
10. Palpate carotid pulse (5–10 seconds): • If present, continue rescue breathing at rate of 12 breaths/min. • If absent, begin external cardiac compressions. *Comments:*	☐	☐	☐	
11. Perform cardiac compressions as follows: • Maintain position on knees parallel to sternum.	☐	☐	☐	

continued on the following page

continued from the previous page

Procedure 32-6 Administering Cardiopulmonary Resuscitation (CPR)	Able to Perform	Able to Perform with Assistance	Unable to Perform	Initials/Date

• Position hands for compressions.
  a. With hand nearest to legs, use index finger to locate lower rib margin and quickly move fingers up to location where ribs connect to sternum.
  b. Place middle finger of this hand on notch where ribs meet sternum and index finger next to it.
  c. Place heel of opposite hand next to index finger on sternum.
  d. Remove first hand from notch and place on top of hand that is on sternum so that they are on top of each other.
  e. Extend or interface fingers and do not allow them to touch chest.
  f. Keep arms straight with shoulders directly over hands on sternum and lock elbows.
  g. Compress adult chest 3.89–5.0 cm (1 1/2–2 inches) at the rate of approximately 100 compressions/min.
  h. Heel of hand must completely release pressure between compressions, but should remain in constant contact with client's skin.
  i. Use the mnemonic "one and, two and, three and..." to keep rhythm and timing.
  j. Ventilate client as described in Action 8.
Comments:				

12. Maintain compression rate for approximately 100 times/min, interjecting 2 ventilations after every 15 compressions. (compression:ventilation rate at 15:2). *Comments:*	☐	☐	☐	

continued on the following page

continued from the previous page

Procedure 32-6 Administering Cardiopulmonary Resuscitation (CPR)	Able to Perform	Able to Perform with Assistance	Unable to Perform	Initials/Date
13. Reassess client after 4 cycles. *Comments:*	☐	☐	☐	
CPR: Two Rescuers—Adult, Adolescent 14. Follow steps above, with following changes: • One rescuer is positioned facing client parallel to head while other rescuer is positioned on opposite side facing client parallel to sternum next to trunk. • Rescuer positioned at client's trunk is responsible for performing cardiac compressions and maintaining verbal mnemonic count. This is rescuer 1. • Rescuer 2 positioned at client's head is responsible for monitoring respirations, assessing carotid pulse, establishing an open airway, and performing rescue breathing. • Maintain compression rate for approximately 100 times/min, interjecting 2 ventilations after every 15 compressions (15:2 ratio). • Rescuer 2 palpates carotid pulse with each chest compression during first full minute. • Rescuer 2 is responsible for calling for a change when fatigued, following this protocol. • Rescuer 1 calls for a change and completes 15 chest compressions. • Rescuer 2 administers 2 breaths and then moves to a position parallel to client's sternum and assumes proper hand position. • Rescuer 1 moves to rescue breathing position and checks carotid pulse for 5 seconds. If cardiac arrest persists, rescuer 1 says, "continue CPR" and delivers one breath. Rescuer 2 resumes cardiac compressions immediately after breath. *Comments:*	☐	☐	☐	

continued on the following page

continued from the previous page

Procedure 32-6 Administering Cardiopulmonary Resuscitation (CPR)	Able to Perform	Able to Perform with Assistance	Unable to Perform	Initials/Date
CPR: One Rescuer—Child (1–7 years) 15. Assess responsiveness, activate emergency medical system, position child, apply appropriate body substance isolation, position self, open airway, and assess for respirations as described in Actions 1–7. *Comments:*	☐	☐	☐	
16. If respirations are absent, begin rescue breathing: • Give two slow breaths (1–1 1/2 sec/breath), pausing to take a breath in between. • Use only amount of air needed to make chest rise. *Comments:*	☐	☐	☐	
17. Palpate carotid pulse (5–10 seconds). If present, ventilate at a rate of once every 4 seconds or 15 times/min. If absent, begin cardiac compressions. *Comments:*	☐	☐	☐	

18. Cardiac compressions (child 1–7 years):
• Maintain position on knees parallel to child's sternum.
• Position hands for compressions.
  a. Locate lower margin of rib cage using hand closest to feet and find notch where ribs and sternum meet.
  b. Place middle finger of this hand on notch and then place index finger next to middle finger.
  c. Place heel of other hand next to index finger of first hand on sternum with heel parallel to sternum (1 cm above the xiphoid process).
	☐	☐	☐	

continued on the following page

continued from the previous page

Procedure 32-6 Administering Cardiopulmonary Resuscitation (CPR)	Able to Perform	Able to Perform with Assistance	Unable to Perform	Initials/Date
d. Keeping elbows locked and shoulders over child, compress sternum 2.5–3.8 cm (1 –1 1/2 inches) at approximate rate of 100 times/min. e. Keep other hand on child's forehead. f. At end of every fifth compression, administer a ventilation (1–1 1/2 seconds). g. Re-evaluate child after 20 cycles. h. A 1-minute CPR should be performed for infants and children up to age 8 before calling 911. In institutions, follow hospital protocol. *Comments:*				
CPR: One Rescuer—Infant (1–12 months) 19. Assess responsiveness, activate emergency medical system, position child, apply appropriate body substance isolation, position self, open airway, and assess for respirations as described in Actions 1–7. *Comments:*	☐	☐	☐	
20. If respirations are absent, begin rescue breathing: • Avoid overextension of infant's neck. • Place a small towel or diaper under infant's shoulders or use a hand to support neck. • Make a tight seal over both infant's nose and mouth and gently administer artificial respirations. • Give two slow breaths (1–1 1/2 sec/breath), pausing to take a breath in between. • Use only amount of air needed to make chest rise. *Comments:*	☐	☐	☐	

continued on the following page

continued from the previous page

Procedure 32-6 Administering Cardiopulmonary Resuscitation (CPR)	Able to Perform	Able to Perform with Assistance	Unable to Perform	Initials/Date
21. Assess circulatory status using brachial pulse: • Locate brachial pulse on inside of upper arm between elbow and shoulder by placing thumb on outside of arm and palpating proximal side of arm with index finger and middle fingers. • If pulse is palpated, continue rescue breathing 20 times/min or once every 3 seconds. • If pulse is absent, begin cardiac compressions. *Comments:*	☐	☐	☐	

22. Cardiac compressions (infant 1–12 months):
• Maintain position parallel to infant.
• Place a small towel or other support under infant's shoulders and neck.
• Position hands for compressions:
  a. Using hand closest to infant's feet, locate intermammary line where it intersects sternum.
  b. Place index finger 1 cm blow this location on sternum and place middle finger next to index finger.
  c. Using these two fingers, compress in a downward motion 1.3–2.5 cm (1/2–1 inch) at rate of 100 times/min.
  d. Keep other hand on infant's forehead.
  e. At end of every fifth compression, administer a ventilation (1–1 1/2 seconds).
  f. Reevaluate infant after 20 cycles.
  g. A 1-minute CPR should be performed for infants and children up to age 8 before calling 911.
Comments:
	☐	☐	☐	

continued on the following page

continued from the previous page

Procedure 32-6 Administering Cardiopulmonary Resuscitation (CPR)	Able to Perform	Able to Perform with Assistance	Unable to Perform	Initials/Date
CPR: Two Rescuers—Child (1–7 years) and Infant (1–12 months) 23. Follow Action 14 for two-rescuer CPR for adults with the following changes: • Utilize child or infant procedure for chest compressions. • Change ratio of compressions to ventilation to 5:1. • Deliver ventilation on upstroke of third compression. *Comments:*	☐	☐	☐	
CPR—Neonate or Premature Infant 24. Follow infant guidelines with the following changes for chest compressions: • Encircle chest with both hands. • Position thumbs over midsternum. • Compress midsternum with both thumbs. • Compress 1.3–1.8 cm (1/2–3/4 inch) at a rate of 100–120 times/min. *Comments:*	☐	☐	☐	
25. If properly trained, use an automated external defibrillator (AED). AED are not recommended for children under 8 years of age. In hospital setting, use defibrillator as specified by institution protocol. *Comments:*	☐	☐	☐	

Checklist for Procedure 33-1   Measuring Intake and Output

Name _____ Date _____

School _____

Instructor _____

Course _____

Procedure 33-1 Measuring Intake and Output	Able to Perform	Able to Perform with Assistance	Unable to Perform	Initials/Date
1. Wash hands/hand hygiene. *Comments:*	☐	☐	☐	
2. Explain rules of I&O record. All fluids taken orally must be recorded on client's intake and output form. • Client must void into bedpan or urinal, not into toilet. • Toilet tissue should be disposed of in plastic-lined container, not in bedpan. *Comments:*	☐	☐	☐	
3. Measure all oral fluids in accord with institution policy. Record all IV fluids as they are infused. *Comments:*	☐	☐	☐	
4. Record time and amount of all fluid intake in designated space on bedside form (oral, tube feedings, IV fluids). *Comments:*	☐	☐	☐	
5. Transfer 8-hour total fluid intake to graphic sheet or 24-hour I&O record on client's chart. *Comments:*	☐	☐	☐	
6. Record all fluid intake in appropriate column of 24-hour record. *Comments:*	☐	☐	☐	

continued on the following page

continued from the previous page

Procedure 33-1 Measuring Intake and Output	Able to Perform	Able to Perform with Assistance	Unable to Perform	Initials/Date
7. Complete 24-hour intake record by adding all 8-hour totals. *Comments:*	☐	☐	☐	
Output 8. Apply nonsterile gloves. *Comments:*	☐	☐	☐	
9. Empty urinal, bedpan, or Foley drainage bag into graduated container or commode hat. *Comments:*	☐	☐	☐	
10. Remove gloves. Wash hands/hand hygiene. *Comments:*	☐	☐	☐	
11. Record time and amount of output (urine, drainage from nasogastric tube, drainage tube) on I&O record. *Comments:*	☐	☐	☐	
12. Transfer 8-hour output totals to graphic sheet or 24-hour I&O record on client's chart. *Comments:*	☐	☐	☐	
13. Complete 24-hour output record by totaling all 8-hour totals. *Comments:*	☐	☐	☐	
14. Wash hands/hand hygiene. *Comments:*	☐	☐	☐	

Checklist for Procedure 33-2   Preparing an IV Solution

Name _____ Date _____

School _____

Instructor _____

Course _____

Procedure 33-2 Preparing an IV Solution	Able to Perform	Able to Perform with Assistance	Unable to Perform	Initials/Date
1. Check prescribing practitioner's order. *Comments:*	☐	☐	☐	
2. Wash hands/hand hygiene. Apply gloves, if needed. *Comments:*	☐	☐	☐	
3. Prepare new bag by removing protective cover from bag. *Comments:*	☐	☐	☐	
4. Inspect bag for leaks, tears, or cracks. Inspect fluid for clarity, particulate matter, and color. Check expiration date. *Comments:*	☐	☐	☐	
5. Prepare label for IV bag: • On label, note date, time, and your initials. • Attach label to bag. Keep in mind bag will be inverted when hanging. Make sure label can be read when IV is hanging. *Comments:*	☐	☐	☐	
6. Store prepared IV solution in area assigned by institution. *Comments:*	☐	☐	☐	

continued on the following page

continued from the previous page

Procedure 33-2 Preparing an IV Solution	Able to Perform	Able to Perform with Assistance	Unable to Perform	Initials/Date
7. Remove gloves and dispose with all used materials. *Comments:*	☐	☐	☐	
8. Wash hands/hand hygiene. *Comments:*	☐	☐	☐	
9. Document procedure. *Comments:*	☐	☐	☐	
Hanging the Prepared IV 10. Wash hands/hand hygiene. *Comments:*	☐	☐	☐	
11. Obtain IV solution for client. Check label on IV bag to ensure matches order. *Comments:*	☐	☐	☐	
12. Inspect bag for leaks, tears, and cracks. Inspect fluid for clarity, particulate matter, and color. *Comments:*	☐	☐	☐	
13. Check client's identification bracelet. *Comments:*	☐	☐	☐	
14. Prepare IV time tape for IV bag: • On time tape, note rate solution is to infuse. • Mark approximate infusion intervals. • Attach time tape to bag. Because bag is inverted, place time tape so can be read when IV is hanging. *Comments:*	☐	☐	☐	

continued on the following page

continued from the previous page

Procedure 33-2 Preparing an IV Solution	Able to Perform	Able to Perform with Assistance	Unable to Perform	Initials/Date
15. Make sure clamp on tubing is closed. Grasp port of IV bag with nondominant hand, remove plastic tab covering the port, and insert full length of spike into bag's port. *Comments:*	☐	☐	☐	
16. Compress drip chamber to fill halfway. *Comments:*	☐	☐	☐	
17. Loosen protective cap from needle or end of IV tubing; open roller clamp and flush tubing with solution. *Comments:*	☐	☐	☐	
18. Close roller clamp and replace cap protector. *Comments:*	☐	☐	☐	
19. When ready to initiate infusion, remove cap protector from tubing. Attach IV tubing to venipuncture catheter. *Comments:*	☐	☐	☐	
20. Open clamp and regulate flow or, if applicable, attach tubing to infusion device or rate controller, if used. Turn on pump and set flow rate. *Comments:*	☐	☐	☐	
21. Wash hands/hand hygiene. *Comments:*	☐	☐	☐	

Checklist for Procedure 33-3 Preparing the IV Bag and Tubing

Name _____ Date _____

School _____

Instructor _____

Course _____

Procedure 33-3 Preparing the IV Bag and Tubing	Able to Perform	Able to Perform with Assistance	Unable to Perform	Initials/Date
1. Check prescribing practitioner's order for IV solution. *Comments:*	☐	☐	☐	
2. Wash hands/hand hygiene. *Comments:*	☐	☐	☐	
3. Check client's identification bracelet. Gather equipment. *Comments:*	☐	☐	☐	
4. Prepare new bag by removing protective cover. Check expiration date on bag and assess for cloudiness or leakage. *Comments:*	☐	☐	☐	
5. Open new infusion set. Unroll tubing and close roller clamp. *Comments:*	☐	☐	☐	
6. Spike bag with tip of new tubing and compress drip chamber to fill halfway. *Comments:*	☐	☐	☐	
7. Open roller clamp, remove protective cap from end of tubing, and slowly flush solution completely through tubing. *Comments:*	☐	☐	☐	

continued on the following page

continued from the previous page

Procedure 33-3 Preparing the IV Bag and Tubing	Able to Perform	Able to Perform with Assistance	Unable to Perform	Initials/Date
8. Close roller clamp and replace cap protector. *Comments:*	☐	☐	☐	
9. Apply clean gloves. *Comments:*	☐	☐	☐	
10. Remove old tubing and replace with new tubing: • Place sterile 2 × 2 gauze under IV catheter or heparin lock. • Stabilize hub of catheter or needle and gently pull out old tubing. • Quickly insert new tubing into catheter hub or needle. • Open roller clamp to establish flow of IV solution. • Reestablish drip rate. • Apply new dressing to IV site. *Comments:*	☐	☐	☐	
11. Discard old tubing and IV bag. *Comments:*	☐	☐	☐	
12. Remove gloves and dispose with all used materials. *Comments:*	☐	☐	☐	
13. Apply a label with date and time of change to tubing. Calculate IV drip rates and begin infusion at prescribed rate. *Comments:*	☐	☐	☐	
14. Wash hands/hand hygiene. *Comments:*	☐	☐	☐	

Checklist for Procedure 33-4 Assessing and Maintaining an IV Insertion Site

Name _____ Date _____

School _____

Instructor _____

Course _____

Procedure 33-4 Assessing and Maintaining an IV Insertion Site	Able to Perform	Able to Perform with Assistance	Unable to Perform	Initials/Date
1. Review prescribing practitioner's order for IV therapy. Comments:	☐	☐	☐	
2. Review client's history for medical conditions or allergies. Comments:	☐	☐	☐	
3. Review client's IV site record and intake and output record. Comments:	☐	☐	☐	
4. Wash hands/hand hygiene. Comments:	☐	☐	☐	
5. Assemble equipment and obtain client's vital signs. Comments:	☐	☐	☐	
6. Check IV fluid for correct fluid, additives, rate, and volume at beginning of shift. Comments:	☐	☐	☐	
7. Check IV tubing for tight connections every 4 hours. Comments:	☐	☐	☐	
8. Check gauze IV dressing hourly to be sure is dry and intact. Comments:	☐	☐	☐	

continued on the following page

continued from the previous page

Procedure 33-4 Assessing and Maintaining an IV Insertion Site	Able to Perform	Able to Perform with Assistance	Unable to Perform	Initials/Date
9. If gauze is not dry and intact, remove dressing and observe site for redness, swelling, or drainage. *Comments:*	☐	☐	☐	
10. If occlusive dressing used, do not remove dressing when assessing site. *Comments:*	☐	☐	☐	
11. Observe vein track for redness, swelling, warmth, or pain hourly. *Comments:*	☐	☐	☐	
12. Document IV site findings in nursing record or flow sheet. *Comments:*	☐	☐	☐	
13. Wash hands/hand hygiene. *Comments:*	☐	☐	☐	

Checklist for Procedure 33-5   Changing the IV Solution

Name _____ Date _____

School _____

Instructor _____

Course _____

Procedure 33-5 Changing the IV Solution	Able to Perform	Able to Perform with Assistance	Unable to Perform	Initials/Date
1. Check prescribing practitioner's order for the IV solution. *Comments:*	☐	☐	☐	
2. Wash hands/hand hygiene. Don clean gloves. *Comments:*	☐	☐	☐	
3. Check client's identification bracelet. *Comments:*	☐	☐	☐	
4. Prepare new bag with additives as ordered by prescribing practitioner. • Prepare bag at least 1 hour before needed. • Change solution when IV bag is empty but there is still solution in drip chamber. *Comments:*	☐	☐	☐	
5. Be sure drip chamber is at least half full. *Comments:*	☐	☐	☐	
6. Change IV solution: • Move roller clamp to stop flow of fluid. • Remove old IV bag from IV pole and hang new bag. • Spike new bag with tubing. • Reestablish flow rate. *Comments:*	☐	☐	☐	

continued on the following page

continued from the previous page

Procedure 33-5 Changing the IV Solution	Able to Perform	Able to Perform with Assistance	Unable to Perform	Initials/Date
7. Check for air in tubing. • If air present, close roller clamp. While stretching tubing, flick tubing with finger and watch bubbles rise to drip chamber. • If large amount of air in tubing, insert needle with empty syringe into port below air and allow air to enter syringe as it flows to client. *Comments:*	☐	☐	☐	
8. Empty remaining fluid from old IV, if needed. *Comments:*	☐	☐	☐	
9. Remove gloves and dispose of all used materials. *Comments:*	☐	☐	☐	
10. Apply label with date, time, and type of solution. *Comments:*	☐	☐	☐	
11. Wash hands/hand hygiene. *Comments:*	☐	☐	☐	

Checklist for Procedure 33-6 Flushing a Central Venous Catheter

Name _____ Date _____

School _____

Instructor _____

Course _____

Procedure 33-6 Flushing a Central Venous Catheter	Able to Perform	Able to Perform with Assistance	Unable to Perform	Initials/Date
1. Wash hands/hand hygiene. Apply gloves, gown, and other protective equipment, as needed. *Comments:*	☐	☐	☐	
2. Prepare two syringes: one with 10 ml normal saline and one with 5 ml heparin solution. *Comments:*	☐	☐	☐	
3. Swab injection cap or catheter hub with povidone-iodine and alcohol. *Comments:*	☐	☐	☐	
4. Clamp catheter and remove cap. *Comments:*	☐	☐	☐	
5. Check catheter for patency: • Attach syringe with normal saline. • Release clamp. • Aspirate heparin solution from catheter. • Observe blood return. • Flush quickly with normal saline. • Reclamp. • Remove empty syringe. • Attach heparin syringe to catheter. • Release clamp. • Flush quickly. • Reclamp. *Comments:*	☐	☐	☐	

continued on the following page

continued from the previous page

Procedure 33-6 Flushing a Central Venous Catheter	Able to Perform	Able to Perform with Assistance	Unable to Perform	Initials/Date
6. Place new cap on end of catheter, tape all tubing connections, and attach tubing to client's clothing. *Comments:*	☐	☐	☐	
7. Dispose of soiled equipment and used supplies. *Comments:*	☐	☐	☐	
8. Wash hands/hand hygiene. *Comments:*	☐	☐	☐	

Checklist for Procedure 33-7   Setting the IV Flow Rate

Name _____   Date _____

School _____

Instructor _____

Course _____

Procedure 33-7 Setting the IV Flow Rate	Able to Perform	Able to Perform with Assistance	Unable to Perform	Initials/Date
1. Check prescribing practitioner's order for IV solution and rate of infusion. *Comments:*	☐	☐	☐	
2. Wash hands/hand hygiene. *Comments:*	☐	☐	☐	
3. Check client's identification bracelet. *Comments:*	☐	☐	☐	
4. Prepare to set flow rate: • Have paper and pencil ready to calculate flow rate. • Review calibration in drops per milliliter of each infusion set. *Comments:*	☐	☐	☐	
5. Determine hourly rate by dividing total volume by total hours. *Comments:*	☐	☐	☐	
6. Mark a length of tape placed on IV bag with hourly time periods, according to rate. *Comments:*	☐	☐	☐	
7. Calculate minute rate based on drop factor of infusion set. *Comments:*	☐	☐	☐	

continued on the following page

continued from the previous page

Procedure 33-7 Setting the IV Flow Rate	Able to Perform	Able to Perform with Assistance	Unable to Perform	Initials/Date
8. Set flow rate using appropriate device: • For regular tubing without a device: Count drops in drip chamber for 1 minute while watching second hand of watch and adjust the roller clamp, as necessary. • For an infusion pump: Insert tubing into flow control chamber, select desired rate (generally calibrated in cc/min), open roller clamp, and push start button. • For a controller: Place IV bag 36 inches above IV site, select desired drops/min, open roller clamp, and count drops for 1 minute to verify rate. • For volume control device: Place device between IV bag and insertion spike of IV tubing, fill with 1–2 hours amount of IV fluid, and count drops for 1 minute. *Comments:*	☐	☐	☐	
9. Monitor infusion rates and IV site for infiltration. *Comments:*	☐	☐	☐	
10. Assess infusion when alarm sounds. *Comments:*	☐	☐	☐	
11. Wash hands/hand hygiene. *Comments:*	☐	☐	☐	

Checklist for Procedure 33-8 Changing the Central Venous Dressing

Name _____ Date _____

School _____

Instructor _____

Course _____

Procedure 33-8 Changing the Central Venous Dressing	Able to Perform	Able to Perform with Assistance	Unable to Perform	Initials/Date
1. Wash hands/hand hygiene; don clean gloves. Open dressing tray. *Comments:*	☐	☐	☐	
2. Remove old dressing carefully, being careful not to dislodge central catheter. *Comments:*	☐	☐	☐	
3. Note drainage on dressing. *Comments:*	☐	☐	☐	
4. Inspect skin at insertion site for redness, tenderness, or swelling. *Comments:*	☐	☐	☐	
5. Palpate tunneled catheter for presence of Dacron cuff, being careful not to palpate close to exit site. *Comments:*	☐	☐	☐	
6. Visually inspect catheter from hub to skin. *Comments:*	☐	☐	☐	
7. Remove gloves and put on sterile gloves. *Comments:*	☐	☐	☐	

continued on the following page

continued from the previous page

Procedure 33-8 Changing the Central Venous Dressing	Able to Perform	Able to Perform with Assistance	Unable to Perform	Initials/Date
8. Clean exit site according to institution protocol. Most use alcohol wipes first, then povidone-iodine swab, beginning at the catheter and moving out in a circular manner for 3 cm to maintain aseptic technique. *Comments:*	☐	☐	☐	
9. Check agency policy about use of ointment to exit site. *Comments:*	☐	☐	☐	
10. Apply transparent dressing. *Comments:*	☐	☐	☐	
11. Label with date and time of dressing change. Gauze dressings changed every 48 hours on peripheral and central catheters. Transparent semipermeable membrane dressings changed at time of access site rotation or every 3–7 days, whichever occurs first. *Comments:*	☐	☐	☐	
12. Secure tubing to client's clothing. *Comments:*	☐	☐	☐	
13. Remove gloves and dispose of all used materials. *Comments:*	☐	☐	☐	
14. Wash hands/hand hygiene. *Comments:*	☐	☐	☐	

Checklist for Procedure 33-9 Discontinuing the IV and Changing to a Saline or Heparin Lock

Name _____ Date _____

School _____

Instructor _____

Course _____

Procedure 33-9 Discontinuing the IV and Changing to a Saline or Heparin Lock	Able to Perform	Able to Perform with Assistance	Unable to Perform	Initials/Date
1. Check prescribing practitioner's order to discontinue IV and insert saline lock. *Comments:*	☐	☐	☐	
2. Wash hands/hand hygiene; don clean gloves. *Comments:*	☐	☐	☐	
3. Check client's identification bracelet. *Comments:*	☐	☐	☐	
4. Explain procedure and reason for discontinuing IV to client. *Comments:*	☐	☐	☐	
5. Prepare supplies at bedside: • Syringe with saline • Syringe with heparin • Saline lock *Comments:*	☐	☐	☐	

continued on the following page

continued from the previous page

Procedure 33-9 Discontinuing the IV and Changing to a Saline or Heparin Lock	Able to Perform	Able to Perform with Assistance	Unable to Perform	Initials/Date
6. If inserting a new saline lock: Prime extension tubing with saline and place saline lock on it. Follow procedures for starting IV, including assessing and preparing site, inserting over-the-needle-catheter (ONC) or butterfly needle, and obtaining a blood return. Do not attach needle or ONC to IV tubing. Instead, attach ONC to extension tubing. Dress site per policy. If inserting new saline lock, prime extension tubing with solution and place connector in hub of angiocatheter. For needleless systems follow steps of manufacturer. In a spring-loaded, retractable needle system, press button after a flashback of blood is observed. To ensure needle separation, turn angiocatheter 360° at hub before inserting the catheter into vein. Advance catheter and attach to extension tubing with addition of a one-way needleless safety valve, which has been flushed with solution. Secure with dressing per institution protocol. *Comments:*	☐	☐	☐	
7. If discontinuing an IV and converting to a saline lock: • Stop IV infusion. • For IV tubing, roll clamp to close IV tubing. • For infusion pump, turn switch to off. *Comments:*	☐	☐	☐	
8. Place saline lock: • Open sterile package with needleless adapter saline lock. • For existing IV, loosen IV tubing and remove. • Screw saline lock into hub of tubing.	☐	☐	☐	

continued on the following page

continued from the previous page

Procedure 33-9 Discontinuing the IV and Changing to a Saline or Heparin Lock	Able to Perform	Able to Perform with Assistance	Unable to Perform	Initials/Date
• To check for patency, remove cap from one-way valve following vigorous scrubbing with alcohol at connection site. Connect needleless Luer-Lok syringe to valve. Inject solution into IV site per protocol, using gentle pulsating motions to create turbulence. Remove syringe and replace sterile cap at end of tubing. *Comments:*				
9. Check for patency of IV: • Clean saline lock with antiseptic solution (usually alcohol wipe). • Insert saline syringe with 25-gauge needle into center of diaphragm. (Needleless system will not require needle.) • Pull back gently on syringe and watch for blood return. • Inject saline slowly into lock. • Assess client's pain at site. *Comments:*	☐	☐	☐	
10. Keep lock patent with heparin or normal saline. Every 8 hours: • Clean rubber diaphragm with antiseptic swab (not applicable if needleless system). • Insert syringe or needleless adapter with heparin or saline into diaphragm. • Inject heparin or saline slowly into lock. *Comments:*	☐	☐	☐	
11. Remove syringe or needleless adapter from diaphragm and swab with antiseptic swab. Discard needle or adapter in sharps container. *Comments:*	☐	☐	☐	

continued on the following page

continued from the previous page

Procedure 33-9 **Discontinuing the IV and Changing to a Saline or Heparin Lock**	**Able to Perform**	**Able to Perform with Assistance**	**Unable to Perform**	**Initials/Date**
12. Assess site for any signs of leakage, irritation, or infiltration. *Comments:*	☐	☐	☐	
13. Remove gloves and dispose with all used materials. *Comments:*	☐	☐	☐	
14. Wash hands/hand hygiene. *Comments:*	☐	☐	☐	

Checklist for Procedure 33-10 Administering a Blood Transfusion

Name _____ Date _____

School _____

Instructor _____

Course _____

Procedure 33-10 Administering a Blood Transfusion	Able to Perform	Able to Perform with Assistance	Unable to Perform	Initials/Date
1. Verify prescribing practitioner's order for transfusion. *Comments:*	☐	☐	☐	
2. If a venipuncture is necessary, refer to Procedure 28-1. *Comments:*	☐	☐	☐	
3. Explain procedure to client. *Comments:*	☐	☐	☐	
4. Review side effects (dyspnea, chills, headache, chest pain, itching) with client and ask client to report these to nurse. *Comments:*	☐	☐	☐	
5. Have client sign consent form. *Comments:*	☐	☐	☐	
6. Obtain baseline vital signs. *Comments:*	☐	☐	☐	
7. Obtain blood product from blood bank within 30 minutes of initiation. *Comments:*	☐	☐	☐	
8. Verify and record blood product and identify client with another nurse. • Client's name, blood group, Rh type • Cross-match compatibility	☐	☐	☐	

continued on the following page

continued from the previous page

Procedure 33-10 Administering a Blood Transfusion	Able to Perform	Able to Perform with Assistance	Unable to Perform	Initials/Date
• Donor blood group and Rh type • Unit and hospital number • Expiration date and time on blood bag • Type of blood product compared with prescribing practitioner's order • Presence of clots in blood *Comments:*				
9. Have client empty bladder. *Comments:*	☐	☐	☐	
10. Wash hands/hand hygiene; put on gloves. *Comments:*	☐	☐	☐	
11. Open blood administration kit and move roller clamps to "off" position. *Comments:*	☐	☐	☐	
12. For Y-tubing, set: • Spike the 0.9% sodium chloride bag and open roller clamp on Y-tubing connected to bag and roller clamp on unused inlet tube until tubing from 0.9% sodium chloride bag is filled. Close clamp on unused tubing. • Squeeze sides of drip chamber and allow filter to partially fill. • Open lower roller clamp and allow tubing to fill with 0.9% sodium chloride. • Close lower clamp. • Invert blood bag once or twice. Spike blood bag and open clamps on inlet tube to allow blood to cover filter completely. • Close lower clamp. *Comments:*	☐	☐	☐	

continued on the following page

continued from the previous page

Procedure 33-10 Administering a Blood Transfusion	Able to Perform	Able to Perform with Assistance	Unable to Perform	Initials/Date
13. For single-tubing set: • Spike blood unit. • Squeeze drip chamber and allow filter to fill with blood. • Open roller clamp and allow tubing to fill with blood to hub. • Prime another IV tubing with 0.9% sodium chloride and piggyback it to blood administration set with a needle; secure all connections with tape. *Comments:*	☐	☐	☐	
14. Attach tubing to venous catheter using sterile precautions and open lower clamp. *Comments:*	☐	☐	☐	
15. Infuse blood at rate of 2–5 ml/min, according to prescribing practitioner's order. *Comments:*	☐	☐	☐	
16. Remain with client for first 15–30 minutes, monitoring vital signs every 5 minutes for 15 minutes, then every 15 minutes for 1 hour, then hourly until 1 hour after infusion is completed, or per institution policy. *Comments:*	☐	☐	☐	
17. After blood has infused, allow tubing to clear with 0.9% sodium chloride. *Comments:*	☐	☐	☐	
18. Appropriately dispose of bloodbag, tubing, and gloves in a biohazard bag and follow policy regarding disposition. Wash hands/hand hygiene. *Comments:*	☐	☐	☐	

continued on the following page

continued from the previous page

Procedure 33-10 Administering a Blood Transfusion	Able to Perform	Able to Perform with Assistance	Unable to Perform	Initials/Date
19. Document procedure. *Comments:*	☐	☐	☐	

Checklist for Procedure 34-1   Inserting a Nasogastric or Nasointestinal Tube for Suction and Enteral Feedings

Name _____ Date _____

School _____

Instructor _____

Course _____

Procedure 34-1 Inserting a Nasogastric or Nasointestinal Tube for Suction and Enteral Feedings	Able to Perform	Able to Perform with Assistance	Unable to Perform	Initials/Date
1. Review client's medical record. *Comments:*	☐	☐	☐	
Nasogastric Tube Insertion 2. Gather equipment. Wash hands/hand hygiene. *Comments:*	☐	☐	☐	
3. Check client's armband; explain procedure, showing items. *Comments:*	☐	☐	☐	
4. Place client in Fowler's position, at least a 45° angle, with pillow behind shoulders; provide for privacy. *Place comatose clients in semi-Fowler's position.* *Comments:*	☐	☐	☐	
5. Place towel over chest, with tissues in reach. Don gloves. *Comments:*	☐	☐	☐	
6. Examine nostrils and assess as client breathes through each nostril. *Comments:*	☐	☐	☐	
7. Measure length of tubing needed, by using tube as a tape measure: • Measure from bridge of client's nose to earlobe to xiphoid process of sternum.	☐	☐	☐	

continued on the following page

continued from the previous page

Procedure 34-1 **Inserting a Nasogastric or Nasointestinal Tube for Suction and Enteral Feedings**	**Able to Perform**	**Able to Perform with Assistance**	**Unable to Perform**	**Initials/Date**
• If tube is to go below stomach, add an additional 15–20 cm. • Place a small piece of tape on tube to mark length. *Comments:*				
8. Have client blow nose; encourage swallowing of water if level of consciousness and treatment plan permit. *Comments:*	☐	☐	☐	
9. Lubricate first 4 inches of tube with water-soluble lubricant. *Comments:*	☐	☐	☐	
10. Insert tube as follows: • Gently pass tube into nostril to back of throat (client may gag); aim tube toward back of throat and down. • When client feels tube in back of throat, use flashlight or penlight to locate tip of tube. • Instruct client to flex head toward chest. • Instruct client to swallow; offer ice chips or water, and advance tube as client swallows. • If resistance is met, rotate tube slowly with downward advancement toward client's closest ear; do not force tube. *Comments:*	☐	☐	☐	
11. Withdraw tube immediately if changes occur in respiratory status. *Comments:*	☐	☐	☐	

continued on the following page

continued from the previous page

Procedure 34-1 **Inserting a Nasogastric or Nasointestinal Tube for Suction and Enteral Feedings**	**Able to Perform**	**Able to Perform with Assistance**	**Unable to Perform**	**Initials/Date**
12. Advance tube, giving client sips of water, until taped mark is reached. *Comments:*	☐	☐	☐	
13. Check placement of tube: • Attach syringe to free end of tube and aspirate sample of gastric contents. Measure with chemstrip pH. • Leave syringe attached to free end of tube. • If prescribed, obtain x-ray; keep client on right side until x-ray is taken. *Comments:*	☐	☐	☐	
14. Secure tube with tape or use a commercially prepared tube holder. • Split 4-inch piece of tape to length of 2 inches and secure tube with tape by placing intact end of tape over bridge of nose. Wrap split ends around tube as exits nose. • Place rubber band, using a slip knot, around exposed tube (12–18 inches from nose toward chest); after x-ray, pin rubber band to client's gown. *Comments:*	☐	☐	☐	
15. Instruct client about movements that dislodge tube. *Comments:*	☐	☐	☐	
16. Gastric decompression: • Remove syringe from free end of tube and connect tube to suction tubing; set machine on type of suction and pressure as prescribed. • Levine tubes are connected to intermittent low pressure. • Salem sump or Anderson's tube is connected to continuous low suction.	☐	☐	☐	

continued on the following page

continued from the previous page

Procedure 34-1 Inserting a Nasogastric or Nasointestinal Tube for Suction and Enteral Feedings	Able to Perform	Able to Perform with Assistance	Unable to Perform	Initials/Date
• Observe nature and amount of gastric tube drainage. • Assess client for nausea, vomiting, and abdominal distention. *Comments:*				
17. Provide oral hygiene and cleanse nares with a tissue. *Comments:*	☐	☐	☐	
18. Remove gloves, dispose of contaminated materials in proper container, and wash hands/hand hygiene. *Comments:*	☐	☐	☐	
19. Position client for comfort, and place call light within easy reach. *Comments:*	☐	☐	☐	
20. Document: • Reason for tube insertion. • Type of tube inserted. • Type of suctioning and pressure setting. • Nature and amount of aspirate and drainage. • Client's tolerance of procedure. • Effectiveness of intervention. *Comments:*	☐	☐	☐	
Insertion of a Small-Bore Feeding Tube 21. Repeat Actions 1–8. *Comments:*	☐	☐	☐	
22. Open adapter cap on tube, snap off end of water vial, and inject water into feeding tube adapter. *Comments:*	☐	☐	☐	

continued on the following page

continued from the previous page

Procedure 34-1 **Inserting a Nasogastric or Nasointestinal Tube for Suction and Enteral Feedings**	Able to Perform	Able to Perform with Assistance	Unable to Perform	Initials/Date
23. Close adapter cap. *Comments:*	☐	☐	☐	
24. Check that stylet does not protrude through holes in feeding tube; adjust, as necessary. *Comments:*	☐	☐	☐	
25. Repeat Actions 9–12. *Comments:*	☐	☐	☐	
26. Check placement of tube: • Aspirate gastric contents with Luer-Lok syringe. • Measure pH of aspirate with chemstrip pH. *Comments:*	☐	☐	☐	
27. Leave stylet in place until x-ray confirms that placement in case tube needs to be advanced into duodenum or jejunum. *Comments:*	☐	☐	☐	
28. Obtain x-ray. Remove stylet from feeding tube after x-ray, and plug open end of tube until feeding. *Comments:*	☐	☐	☐	
29. Repeat Actions 17–20. *Comments:*	☐	☐	☐	
30. Replace small bore tube every 3–4 weeks. *Comments:*	☐	☐	☐	

continued on the following page

continued from the previous page

Procedure 34-1 Inserting a Nasogastric or Nasointestinal Tube for Suction and Enteral Feedings	Able to Perform	Able to Perform with Assistance	Unable to Perform	Initials/Date
31. Wash hands/hand hygiene. *Comments:*	☐	☐	☐	

Checklist for Procedure 34-2   Administering Enteral Tube Feedings

Name _____ Date _____

School _____

Instructor _____

Course _____

Procedure 34-2 Administering Enteral Tube Feedings	Able to Perform	Able to Perform with Assistance	Unable to Perform	Initials/Date
1. Identify client. Review medical record for formula type, amount, and time. *Comments:*	☐	☐	☐	
2. Wash hands/hand hygiene. *Comments:*	☐	☐	☐	
3. Check client's armband. *Comments:*	☐	☐	☐	
4. Explain procedure to client. *Comments:*	☐	☐	☐	
5. Assemble equipment. Add color to formula per institutional policy. If using bag, fill with prescribed amount of formula. *Comments:*	☐	☐	☐	
6. Place client on right side in high Fowler's position. *Comments:*	☐	☐	☐	
7. Wash hands/hand hygiene; don nonsterile gloves. *Comments:*	☐	☐	☐	
8. Provide for privacy. *Comments:*	☐	☐	☐	

continued on the following page

continued from the previous page

Procedure 34-2 Administering Enteral Tube Feedings	Able to Perform	Able to Perform with Assistance	Unable to Perform	Initials/Date
9. Observe for abdominal distention; auscultate for bowel sounds. *Comments:*	☐	☐	☐	
10. Check feeding tube. Insert syringe into adapter port, aspirate stomach contents, and check amount of residue. If residue is greater than 50–100 ml (or according to protocol), hold feeding until residue diminishes. Instill aspirated contents back into feeding tube. *Comments:*	☐	☐	☐	
11. Administer tube feeding. *Comments:*	☐	☐	☐	
Intermittent Bolus 12. Pinch tubing. *Comments:*	☐	☐	☐	
13. Remove plunger from barrel of syringe and attach to adapter. *Comments:*	☐	☐	☐	
14. Fill syringe with formula. *Comments:*	☐	☐	☐	
15. Allow formula to infuse slowly; continue adding formula to syringe until prescribed amount infused. *Comments:*	☐	☐	☐	
16. Flush tubing with 30–60 ml or prescribed amount of water. *Comments:*	☐	☐	☐	

continued on the following page

continued from the previous page

Procedure 34-2 Administering Enteral Tube Feedings	Able to Perform	Able to Perform with Assistance	Unable to Perform	Initials/Date
Intermittent Gavage Feeding 17. Hang bag on IV pole 18 inches above client's head. *Comments:*	☐	☐	☐	
18. Remove air from bag's tubing. *Comments:*	☐	☐	☐	
19. Attach distal end of tubing to feeding tube adapter; adjust drip to infuse over prescribed time. *Comments:*	☐	☐	☐	
20. When bag empties of formula, add 30–60 ml or prescribed amount of water; close clamp. *Comments:*	☐	☐	☐	
21. Change bags every 24 hours. *Comments:*	☐	☐	☐	
Continuous Gavage 22. Check tube placement at least every 4 hours. *Comments:*	☐	☐	☐	
23. Check residual at least every 8 hours. *Comments:*	☐	☐	☐	
24. If residual is above 100 ml, stop feeding. *Comments:*	☐	☐	☐	

continued on the following page

continued from the previous page

Procedure 34-2 Administering Enteral Tube Feedings	Able to Perform	Able to Perform with Assistance	Unable to Perform	Initials/Date
25. Add prescribed amount of formula to bag for a 4-hour period; dilute with water, if prescribed. *Comments:*	☐	☐	☐	
26. Hang gavage bag on IV pole. Prime tubing. *Comments:*	☐	☐	☐	
27. Thread tubing through feeding pump and attach distal end of tubing to feeding tube adapter; keep tubing straight between bag and pump. *Comments:*	☐	☐	☐	
28. Adjust drip rate. *Comments:*	☐	☐	☐	
29. Monitor infusion rate and signs of respiratory distress or diarrhea. *Comments:*	☐	☐	☐	
30. Flush tube with water every 4 hours, as prescribed, or following administration of medications. *Comments:*	☐	☐	☐	
31. Replace disposable feeding bag at least every 24 hours, in accordance with institution's protocol. *Comments:*	☐	☐	☐	
32. Elevate head of bed at least 30° at all times and turn client every 2 hours. *Comments:*	☐	☐	☐	

continued on the following page

continued from the previous page

Procedure 34-2 **Administering Enteral Tube Feedings**	**Able to Perform**	**Able to Perform with Assistance**	**Unable to Perform**	**Initials/Date**
33. Provide oral hygiene every 2–4 hours. *Comments:*	☐	☐	☐	
34. Administer water, as prescribed, with and between feedings. *Comments:*	☐	☐	☐	
35. Remove gloves. Wash hands/hand hygiene. *Comments:*	☐	☐	☐	
36. Record total amount of formula and water administered on I&O form and client's response to feeding. *Comments:*	☐	☐	☐	

Checklist for Procedure 35-1   Administering Patient-Controlled Analgesia (PCA)

Name _____ Date _____

School _____

Instructor _____

Course _____

Procedure 35-1 Administering Patient-Controlled Analgesia (PCA)	Able to Perform	Able to Perform with Assistance	Unable to Perform	Initials/Date
1. Wash hands/hand hygiene. *Comments:*	☐	☐	☐	
2. Assess client's comfort level: pain location, intensity, characteristics, pattern, factors that increase or decrease pain. *Comments:*	☐	☐	☐	
3. Assess client's consciousness level and ability to understand. *Comments:*	☐	☐	☐	
4. Check PCA order for drug, concentration, route, basal infusion rate, bolus dose, lockout interval, maximal dose, and any loading dose. *Comments:*	☐	☐	☐	
5. Check PCA medication label against prescribing practitioner's order and follow "five rights" principle. Medication usually has been placed in PCA syringe in pharmacy. *Comments:*	☐	☐	☐	
6. Read manufacturer's instructions before assembling and programming PCA pump. *Comments:*	☐	☐	☐	

continued on the following page

continued from the previous page

Procedure 35-1 **Administering Patient-Controlled Analgesia (PCA)**	Able to Perform	Able to Perform with Assistance	Unable to Perform	Initials/Date
7. Place filled PCA syringe into chamber in PCA pump and detect any leaking or damage to system. *Comments:*	☐	☐	☐	
8. Program pump according to prescribed parameters, usually including basal infusion rate (mg/hr), bolus dose (mg), lockout interval (min), and maximal dose limit (mg/hr). *Comments:*	☐	☐	☐	
9. Wear gloves. *Comments:*	☐	☐	☐	
10. Inspect existing infusion line and puncture site for any inflammation sign. Check for occlusion or leakage of infusion line. Check IV catheterization or epidural catheter placement if client needs infusion line. *Comments:*	☐	☐	☐	
11. Prime PCA pump tubing. Connect pump tubing with infusion line, using aseptic technique, and secure with adhesive tape. *Comments:*	☐	☐	☐	
12. Give client control button. Instruct how and when to press button. *Comments:*	☐	☐	☐	

continued on the following page

continued from the previous page

Procedure 35-1 **Administering Patient-Controlled Analgesia (PCA)**	**Able to Perform**	**Able to Perform with Assistance**	**Unable to Perform**	**Initials/Date**
13. Record procedure, including start time, type of medication, route, concentration and volume prepared, dosage, loading dose, basal rate, lock-out interval, and maximal dose. *Comments:*	☐	☐	☐	
14. Wash hands/hand hygiene. *Comments:*	☐	☐	☐	

Checklist for Procedure 35-2 Administering Epidural Analgesia

Name _____ Date _____

School _____

Instructor _____

Course _____

Procedure 35-2 Administering Epidural Analgesia	Able to Perform	Able to Perform with Assistance	Unable to Perform	Initials/Date
1. Wash hands/hand hygiene. *Comments:*	☐	☐	☐	
2. Verify medication with order. *Comments:*	☐	☐	☐	
3. Gather equipment needed and verify client's identification. *Comments:*	☐	☐	☐	
4. Set up sterile field. *Comments:*	☐	☐	☐	
For Bolus Injection 5. For bolus injection, draw up prediluted, preservative-free narcotic solution through filter needle in 10-cc syringe. *Comments:*	☐	☐	☐	
6. Change from filter needle to regular 20-gauge needle or needleless system, if in use. *Comments:*	☐	☐	☐	
7. Clean injection cap with povidone-iodine. *Comments:*	☐	☐	☐	

continued on the following page

continued from the previous page

Procedure 35-2 Administering Epidural Analgesia	Able to Perform	Able to Perform with Assistance	Unable to Perform	Initials/Date
8. Insert safety needle into injection cap and aspirate. *Comments:*	☐	☐	☐	
9. If 0.5 cc or less clear fluid returns, inject drug slowly. Assess vital signs before and after administration. *Comments:*	☐	☐	☐	
10. Remove needle from the injection cap and dispose of properly. *Comments:*	☐	☐	☐	
For Continuous Infusion 11. For continuous infusion, attach preservative-free opioid to infusion pump tubing and prime tubing. *Comments:*	☐	☐	☐	
12. Attach proximal end of tubing to pump and distal end to catheter. Luer-Lok all connections. Tape a tension loop of tubing to client's body. Start pump. *Comments:*	☐	☐	☐	
13. Ensure pump is infusing at desired rate. *Comments:*	☐	☐	☐	
14. Label tubing as epidural catheter tubing and with name of drug, date, and time. *Comments:*	☐	☐	☐	
15. Dispose of gloves. Wash hands/hand hygiene. *Comments:*	☐	☐	☐	

continued on the following page

continued from the previous page

Procedure 35-2 Administering Epidural Analgesia	Able to Perform	Able to Perform with Assistance	Unable to Perform	Initials/Date
16. Document in client's chart. *Comments:*	☐	☐	☐	

Checklist for Procedure 36-1   Proper Body Mechanics, Safe Lifting, and Transferring

Name _____ Date _____

School _____

Instructor _____

Course _____

Procedure 36-1 Proper Body Mechanics, Safe Lifting, and Transferring	Able to Perform	Able to Perform with Assistance	Unable to Perform	Initials/Date
1. Wash hands/hygiene. *Comments:*	☐	☐	☐	
2. Assess for obstacles, heavy clients, poor handholds, equipment or objects in the way. Reduce or remove hazards before lifting client or object. Assess for tubing or equipment connected to client. *Comments:*	☐	☐	☐	
3. Assess for slippery surfaces, including wet floors; slippery shoes on client, helper, or nurse; and towels, linen, or paper on floor. Resolve slippery surface before lifting the client or object. *Comments:*	☐	☐	☐	
4. Assess for hidden risks, including client confusion, combativeness, orthostatic hypotension, drug effects, pain, or fear. *Comments:*	☐	☐	☐	
5. Maintain low center of gravity by bending at hips and knees. Squat down rather than bend over to lift and lower the client. *Comments:*	☐	☐	☐	
6. Establish a wide support base with feet spread apart. *Comments:*	☐	☐	☐	

continued on the following page

continued from the previous page

Procedure 36-1 Proper Body Mechanics, Safe Lifting, and Transferring	Able to Perform	Able to Perform with Assistance	Unable to Perform	Initials/Date
7. Use feet to move, not a twisting or bending motion from the waist. *Comments:*	☐	☐	☐	
8. When pushing or pulling: • Stand near object • Stagger one foot partially ahead of the other. *Comments:*	☐	☐	☐	
9. When pushing: • Lean into the client or object and apply continuous light pressure. • Lean away and grasp with light pressure. • Never jerk or twist your body to force a weight to move. *Comments:*	☐	☐	☐	
10. When stooping to move an object: • Maintain a wide base of support with feet. • Flex knees to lower body. • Maintain straight upper body. *Comments:*	☐	☐	☐	
11. When lifting or carrying an object: • Bend the knees in front of the object. • Take a firm hold, and assume a standing position by using leg muscles and keeping back straight. *Comments:*	☐	☐	☐	
12. When rising up from a squatting position: • Arch your back slightly. • Keep the buttocks and abdomen tucked in. • Rise up with your head first. *Comments:*	☐	☐	☐	

continued on the following page

continued from the previous page

Procedure 36-1 **Proper Body Mechanics, Safe Lifting, and Transferring**	**Able to Perform**	**Able to Perform with Assistance**	**Unable to Perform**	**Initials/Date**
13. When lifting or carrying heavy objects, keep weight as close to your center of gravity as possible. *Comments:*	☐	☐	☐	
14. When reaching for a client or an object: • Keep the back straight. • If client or object is heavy, do not try to lift without repositioning yourself closer to the weight. *Comments:*	☐	☐	☐	
15. Use safety aids and equipment. • Use gait belts, lifts, draw sheets, and other transfer assistance devices. • Encourage clients to use handrails and grab bars. • Wheelchair, cart, and stretcher wheels should be locked when they are not being moved. *Comments:*	☐	☐	☐	
16. Wash hands/hand hygiene. *Comments:*	☐	☐	☐	

Checklist for Procedure 36-2   Administering Passive Range-of-Motion (ROM) Exercises

Name _____ Date _____

School _____

Instructor _____

Course _____

Procedure 36-2 Administering Passive Range-of-Motion (ROM) Exercises	Able to Perform	Able to Perform with Assistance	Unable to Perform	Initials/Date
1. Hand hygiene. Wear gloves if contact with body fluids is possible. *Comments:*	☐	☐	☐	
2. Explain procedure to client, including estimated duration. *Comments:*	☐	☐	☐	
3. Provide for privacy, including exposing only the extremity to be exercised. *Comments:*	☐	☐	☐	
4. Adjust bed to comfortable height for performing ROM. *Comments:*	☐	☐	☐	
5. Lower bed rail only on side where you are working. *Comments:*	☐	☐	☐	
6. Describe passive ROM exercises, or verbally cue client to perform ROM exercises with assistance. *Comments:*	☐	☐	☐	
7. Start at client's head and perform ROM exercises down each side of body. *Comments:*	☐	☐	☐	

continued on the following page

continued from the previous page

Procedure 36-2 **Administering Passive Range-of-Motion (ROM) Exercises**	**Able to Perform**	**Able to Perform with Assistance**	**Unable to Perform**	**Initials/Date**
8. Repeat each ROM exercise as client tolerates, to maximum of 5 times. Perform each motion in slow, firm manner. Encourage full joint movement, but do not go beyond point of pain, resistance, or fatigue. *Comments:*	☐	☐	☐	
9. Head: Perform with client in sitting position, if possible. • Rotation: Turn the head from side to side. • Flexion and extension: Tilt the head toward chest and then tilt slightly upward. • Lateral flexion: Tilt head on each side to almost touch ear to shoulder. *Comments:*	☐	☐	☐	
10. Neck: Perform with client in sitting position, if possible. • Rotation: Rotate neck in semicircle while supporting head. *Comments:*	☐	☐	☐	
11. Trunk: Perform with client in sitting position, if possible. • Flexion and extension: Bend trunk forward, straighten trunk, and then extend slightly backward. • Rotation: Turn shoulders forward and return to normal position. Lateral flexion: Tip trunk to left side, straighten trunk, tip to right side. *Comments:*	☐	☐	☐	

continued on the following page

continued from the previous page

Procedure 36-2 **Administering Passive Range-of-Motion (ROM) Exercises**	**Able to Perform**	**Able to Perform with Assistance**	**Unable to Perform**	**Initials/Date**
12. Arm: • Flexion and extension: Extend client's arm in straight position upward toward head, then downward along side. • Adduction and abduction: Extend arm in straight position toward midline (adduction) and away from midline (abduction). *Comments:*	☐	☐	☐	
13. Shoulder: • Internal and external rotation: Bend client's elbow at 90° angle with upper arm parallel to shoulder; rotate shoulder by moving lower arm upward and downward. *Comments:*	☐	☐	☐	
14. Elbow: • Flexion and extension: Supporting arm, flex and extend client's elbow. • Pronation and supination: Flex elbow, move hand in palm-up and palm-down position. *Comments:*	☐	☐	☐	
15. Wrist: • Flexion and extension: Supporting client's wrist, flex and extend wrist. • Adduction and abduction: Supporting lower arm, turn wrist right to left, left to right, then rotate wrist in circular motion. *Comments:*	☐	☐	☐	
16. Hand: • Flexion and extension: Supporting client's wrist, flex and extend fingers. • Adduction and abduction: Supporting wrist, spread fingers apart and then bring them close together.	☐	☐	☐	

continued on the following page

continued from the previous page

Procedure 36-2 Administering Passive Range-of-Motion (ROM) Exercises	Able to Perform	Able to Perform with Assistance	Unable to Perform	Initials/Date
• Opposition: Supporting wrist, touch each finger with tip of thumb. • Thumb rotation: Supporting wrist, rotate thumb in circular manner. *Comments:*				
17. Hip and leg: Perform with client in supine position, if possible. • Flexion and extension: Supporting lower leg, flex leg toward chest and then extend leg. • Internal and external rotation: Supporting lower leg, angle foot inward and outward. *Comments:*	☐	☐	☐	
18. Knee: • Flexion and extension: Supporting client's lower leg, flex and extend knee. *Comments:*	☐	☐	☐	
19. Ankle: • Flexion and extension: Supporting client's lower leg, flex and extend ankle. *Comments:*	☐	☐	☐	
20. Foot: • Adduction and abduction: Supporting client's ankle, spread toes apart and then bring toes close together. • Flexion and extension: Supporting ankle, extend toes upward and then flex toes downward. *Comments:*	☐	☐	☐	

continued on the following page

continued from the previous page

Procedure 36-2 Administering Passive Range-of-Motion (ROM) Exercises	Able to Perform	Able to Perform with Assistance	Unable to Perform	Initials/Date
21. Observe client's joints and face for signs of exertion, pain, or fatigue during movement. *Comments:*	☐	☐	☐	
22. Replace covers and position client in proper body alignment. *Comments:*	☐	☐	☐	
23. Place side rails in upright position. *Comments:*	☐	☐	☐	
24. Place call light within reach. *Comments:*	☐	☐	☐	
25. Hand hygiene. *Comments:*	☐	☐	☐	

Checklist for Procedure 36-3   Turning and Positioning a Client

Name _____ Date _____

School _____

Instructor _____

Course _____

Procedure 36-3 Turning and Positioning a Client	Able to Perform	Able to Perform with Assistance	Unable to Perform	Initials/Date
1. Wash hands/hand hygiene. *Comments:*	☐	☐	☐	
2. Explain procedure to client. Elicit client cooperation and participation. *Comments:*	☐	☐	☐	
3. Gather all necessary equipment. Provide for client privacy. *Comments:*	☐	☐	☐	
4. Secure adequate assistance to complete task safely. *Comments:*	☐	☐	☐	
5. Adjust bed to comfortable working height. Lower side rail on side of bed closest to you. *Comments:*	☐	☐	☐	
6. Follow proper body mechanics guidelines: • When moving client in bed, position bed so that your legs are slightly bent at knees and hips. • Maintain natural curves in your back while lifting. • Position one foot slightly in front of other and spread feet apart to create a wide base for balance. • When arms are placed under client, slowly lean backward onto your back leg using your body weight to help you lift client to one side of bed.	☐	☐	☐	

continued on the following page

continued from the previous page

Procedure 36-3 Turning and Positioning a Client	Able to Perform	Able to Perform with Assistance	Unable to Perform	Initials/Date
• Do not extend or rotate your back to move a client in bed. • If you cannot move client easily, always ask for and obtain assistance for the safety of both you and the client. • Be sure floor is not slippery and that bed is locked. • Always use a turning sheet when rolling a client because this gives you better support and control of client. *Comments:*				
7. Position drains, tubes, and IVs to accommodate client's new position. *Comments:*	☐	☐	☐	
8. Place or assist client into appropriate starting position. Monitor client status, and provide adequate rest breaks or support as necessary. *Comments:*	☐	☐	☐	

Moving from Supine to Side-Lying Position
9. Move client from supine to side-lying position:
• Slide your hands underneath client.
• Move client to one side of bed by lifting client's body toward you in stages:
  • First the upper trunk;
  • Then the lower trunk;
  • Finally, the legs
• Lift client's body; do not drag client across sheets.
• Roll client to side-lying position by placing client's inside arm next to client's body with palm of hand against hip.
• Cross client's outside arm and leg toward midline and logroll client toward you.
	☐	☐	☐	

continued on the following page

continued from the previous page

Procedure 36-3 Turning and Positioning a Client	Able to Perform	Able to Perform with Assistance	Unable to Perform	Initials/Date
• Use client's outside shoulder and hip for leverage while maintaining stability and control of top arm and leg. *Comments:*				
Maintaining Side-Lying Position 10. Repeat Actions 1–8. *Comments:*	☐	☐	☐	
11. Use pillows to support client: • Place to support client's head and arms. • Can be used under topside leg, thigh, knee, ankle, and foot. • Move lower arm forward slightly at shoulder and bend elbow for comfort. • If client is unstable, placing a pillow against the back will provide additional support and keep the client from rolling supine. *Comments:*	☐	☐	☐	
Moving from Side-Lying to Prone Position 12. Repeat Actions 1–8. *Comments:*	☐	☐	☐	
13. To move to prone position: • Remove positioning towels, pillows, or other support devices. • Assess if client's position needs to be adjusted to accommodate continued movement into prone position. • Move client's inside arm next to client's body with palm against hip. • Roll client onto stomach using shoulder and hip as key points of control. • Place the head in a comfortable position to one side without excessive pressure to sensitive areas.	☐	☐	☐	

continued on the following page

continued from the previous page

Procedure 36-3 Turning and Positioning a Client	Able to Perform	Able to Perform with Assistance	Unable to Perform	Initials/Date
• Place pillows under trunk, as needed, to relieve pressure and increase comfort. • Place arms comfortably at client's side and uncross legs with feet approximately a foot apart. *Comments:*				
Maintaining Prone Position 14. To maintain prone: • Use a shallow pillow or folded towel to support client's head comfortably. • Place pillow under abdomen to support back. • Place an additional pillow under lower leg to reduce pressure of toes and forefoot against bed. *Comments:*	☐	☐	☐	
Moving from Prone to Supine Position 15. Repeat Actions 1–8. *Comments:*	☐	☐	☐	
16. To move from prone to supine: • Remove positioning towels or pillows. • Slide your hands underneath client. • Move client segmentally to one side of the bed to accommodate the new position. • Position inside arm next to client's body with client's palm next to hip. • Roll client to supine position by logrolling the client toward you using the client's outside shoulder and hip for leverage. • Position client away from direction of roll to prevent undue pressure. • When client reaches supine, uncross the arms and legs and place into anatomic positions. *Comments:*	☐	☐	☐	

continued on the following page

continued from the previous page

Procedure 36-3 Turning and Positioning a Client	Able to Perform	Able to Perform with Assistance	Unable to Perform	Initials/Date

Maintaining Supine Position
17. To maintain supine position:
   • Use a footboard to support the foot.
   • Use heel protectors or place a pillow between the heel and gastrocnemius muscle to reduce the pressure on the heels.
   • Assess and compare warmth, sensation, color, and movement of feet.
   • Use a trochanter roll to prevent excessive external rotation of the lower extremity.
   • For comfort, place additional pillows to support client's head, arms, or lower back.
Comments:
	☐	☐	☐	

18. Place side rails in upright position. Return bed to low position. *Comments:*	☐	☐	☐	
19. Place call light within reach. *Comments:*	☐	☐	☐	
20. Move bedside table close. Place items of frequent use within reach. *Comments:*	☐	☐	☐	
21. Wash hands/hand hygiene. *Comments:*	☐	☐	☐	

Checklist for Procedure 36-4   Moving a Client in Bed

Name _____ Date _____

School _____

Instructor _____

Course _____

Procedure 36-4 Moving a Client in Bed	Able to Perform	Able to Perform with Assistance	Unable to Perform	Initials/Date
Moving a Client up in Bed with One Nurse 1. Wash hands/hand hygiene. *Comments:*	☐	☐	☐	
2. Inform client of reason for the move and how to assist. *Comments:*	☐	☐	☐	
3. Elevate bed to just below waist height. Lower head of bed, if tolerated. Lower side rails on your side. *Comments:*	☐	☐	☐	
4. Remove the pillow. Place against headboard. *Comments:*	☐	☐	☐	
5. Have client fold arms across chest. *Comments:*	☐	☐	☐	
6. Have client hold on to overhead trapeze, if available. *Comments:*	☐	☐	☐	
7. Have client bend knees and place feet flat on bed. *Comments:*	☐	☐	☐	

continued on the following page

continued from the previous page

Procedure 36-4 Moving a Client in Bed	Able to Perform	Able to Perform with Assistance	Unable to Perform	Initials/Date
8. Stand at an angle to head of bed with feet apart, facing head of bed, and knees bent. *Comments:*	☐	☐	☐	
9. Slide one hand and arm under client's shoulder, the other under client's thigh. *Comments:*	☐	☐	☐	
10. Rock forward toward head of bed, lifting client with you. Have client push with legs. *Comments:*	☐	☐	☐	
11. If client has trapeze, have client pull up holding onto trapeze as you move client upward. *Comments:*	☐	☐	☐	
12. Repeat these steps until client is moved up high enough in bed. *Comments:*	☐	☐	☐	
13. Return client's pillow under the head. *Comments:*	☐	☐	☐	
14. Elevate head of bed, if tolerated by client. *Comments:*	☐	☐	☐	
15. Assess client for comfort. *Comments:*	☐	☐	☐	

continued on the following page

continued from the previous page

Procedure 36-4 Moving a Client in Bed	Able to Perform	Able to Perform with Assistance	Unable to Perform	Initials/Date
16. Adjust the client's bedclothes as needed for comfort. *Comments:*	☐	☐	☐	
17. Lower bed and elevate side rails. *Comments:*	☐	☐	☐	
18. Hand hygiene. *Comments:*	☐	☐	☐	
Moving a Client up in Bed with Two or More Nurses 19. Hand hygiene. *Comments:*	☐	☐	☐	
20. Inform client of reason for the move and how to assist. *Comments:*	☐	☐	☐	
21. Elevate bed to just below waist height. Lower head of bed if tolerated by client. Lower side rails. *Comments:*	☐	☐	☐	
22. With two nurses, place turn or draw sheet under client's back and head. *Comments:*	☐	☐	☐	
23. Roll up draw sheet on each side until it is next to client. *Comments:*	☐	☐	☐	
24. Follow Actions 4–7. *Comments:*	☐	☐	☐	

continued on the following page

continued from the previous page

Procedure 36-4 Moving a Client in Bed	Able to Perform	Able to Perform with Assistance	Unable to Perform	Initials/Date
25. The nurses stand on either side of bed, at an angle to head of bed, with knees flexed and feet apart in wide stance. *Comments:*	☐	☐	☐	
26. The nurses hold their elbows as close as possible to their bodies. *Comments:*	☐	☐	☐	
27. The lead nurse will give signal to move: 1-2-3 go. The nurses will lift up (off of bed) on turn or draw sheet and forward (toward head of bed) in one smooth motion. The move is coordinated to transfer client toward head of bed. Simultaneously, have client push with legs or pull using trapeze. *Comments:*	☐	☐	☐	
28. Repeat until client is moved upright enough in bed to be comfortable. *Comments:*	☐	☐	☐	
29. Return client's pillow under head. *Comments:*	☐	☐	☐	
30. Elevate head of bed, if tolerated by client. *Comments:*	☐	☐	☐	
31. Assess client for comfort. *Comments:*	☐	☐	☐	
32. Adjust client's bedclothes for comfort. *Comments:*	☐	☐	☐	

continued on the following page

continued from the previous page

Procedure 36-4 Moving a Client in Bed	Able to Perform	Able to Perform with Assistance	Unable to Perform	Initials/Date
33. Lower bed and elevate side rails. *Comments:*	☐	☐	☐	
34. Wash hands/hand hygiene. *Comments:*	☐	☐	☐	

Checklist for Procedure 36-5   Assisting from Bed to Wheelchair, Commode, or Chair

Name _____ Date _____

School _____

Instructor _____

Course _____

Procedure 36-5 Assisting from Bed to Wheelchair, Commode, or Chair	Able to Perform	Able to Perform with Assistance	Unable to Perform	Initials/Date
1. Inform client about desired purpose and destination. *Comments:*	☐	☐	☐	
2. Assess client for ability to assist with transfer and presence of cognitive or sensory deficits. *Comments:*	☐	☐	☐	
3. Lock bed in position. Hand hygiene. *Comments:*	☐	☐	☐	
4. Place any splints, braces, or other devices on client. *Comments:*	☐	☐	☐	
5. Place shoes or slippers on client's feet. *Comments:*	☐	☐	☐	
6. Lower height of bed to lowest possible position. *Comments:*	☐	☐	☐	
7. Slowly raise head of bed if not contraindicated by client's condition. *Comments:*	☐	☐	☐	

continued on the following page

continued from the previous page

Procedure 36-5 **Assisting from Bed to Wheelchair, Commode, or Chair**	**Able to Perform**	**Able to Perform with Assistance**	**Unable to Perform**	**Initials/Date**
8. Place one arm under client's legs and one arm behind client's back. Slowly pivot client so client's legs are dangling over edge of bed and client is in a sitting position on edge of bed. *Comments:*	☐	☐	☐	
9. Allow client to dangle for 2 to 5 minutes. Help support client, if necessary. *Comments:*	☐	☐	☐	
10. Bring chair or wheelchair close to side of bed. Place at a 45° angle to bed. If client has a weaker side, place chair or wheelchair on client's strong side. *Comments:*	☐	☐	☐	
11. Lock wheelchair brakes and elevate foot pedals. For chairs, lock brakes, if available. *Comments:*	☐	☐	☐	
12. If using a gait belt to assist client, place it around client's waist. *Comments:*	☐	☐	☐	
13. Assist client to side of bed until feet are firmly on floor and slightly apart. *Comments:*	☐	☐	☐	
14. Grasp sides of gait belt or place your hands just below client's axilla. Using a wide stance, bend your knees and assist client to standing position. *Comments:*	☐	☐	☐	

continued on the following page

continued from the previous page

Procedure 36-5 **Assisting from Bed to Wheelchair, Commode, or Chair**	**Able to Perform**	**Able to Perform with Assistance**	**Unable to Perform**	**Initials/Date**
15. Stand close to client, pivot until client's back is toward chair. *Comments:*	☐	☐	☐	
16. Instruct client to place hands on arm supports or place client's hands on arm supports of chair. *Comments:*	☐	☐	☐	
17. Bend at knees and ease client into a sitting position. *Comments:*	☐	☐	☐	
18. Assist client to maintain proper posture. Support weak side with pillow, if needed. *Comments:*	☐	☐	☐	
19. Secure safety belt, place client's feet on feet pedals, and release brakes if moving client immediately. Make sure tubes and lines, arms, and hands are not pinched or caught between client and chair. If client is sitting in chair, offer a footstool, if available. *Comments:*	☐	☐	☐	
20. Wash hands/hand hygiene. *Comments:*	☐	☐	☐	

Checklist for Procedure 36-6 Assisting from Bed to Stretcher

Name _____ Date _____

School _____

Instructor _____

Course _____

Procedure 36-6 Assisting from Bed to Stretcher	Able to Perform	Able to Perform with Assistance	Unable to Perform	Initials/Date
Transferring a Client with Minimum Assistance 1. Inform client about desired purpose and destination. Hand hygiene. *Comments:*	☐	☐	☐	
2. Raise the height of bed to 1 inch higher than the stretcher and lock brakes of bed. *Comments:*	☐	☐	☐	
3. Instruct client to move to side of bed close to stretcher. Lower side rails of bed and stretcher. Leave side rails on opposite side up. *Comments:*	☐	☐	☐	
4. Stand at outer side of stretcher and push it toward bed. *Comments:*	☐	☐	☐	
5. Instruct client to move onto stretcher providing assistance, as needed. *Comments:*	☐	☐	☐	
6. Cover client with sheet or bath blanket. *Comments:*	☐	☐	☐	
7. Elevate side rails on stretcher and secure safety belts about client. Release brakes of stretcher. *Comments:*	☐	☐	☐	

continued on the following page

continued from the previous page

Procedure 36-6 Assisting from Bed to Stretcher	Able to Perform	Able to Perform with Assistance	Unable to Perform	Initials/Date
8. Stand at head of stretcher to guide it when pushing. *Comments:*	☐	☐	☐	
9. Hand hygiene. *Comments:*	☐	☐	☐	
Transferring a Client with Maximum Assistance 10. Repeat Actions 1 and 2. *Comments:*	☐	☐	☐	
11. Assess amount of assistance required for transfer. Usually 2 to 4 staff members are required for maximally assisted transfer. *Comments:*	☐	☐	☐	
12. Lock wheels of bed and stretcher. *Comments:*	☐	☐	☐	
13. Have one nurse stand close to client's head. *Comments:*	☐	☐	☐	
14. Logroll client (keep in straight alignment) and place a lift sheet under client's back, trunk, and upper legs. The lift sheet can extend under head if client lacks head control abilities. *Comments:*	☐	☐	☐	

continued on the following page

continued from the previous page

Procedure 36-6 Assisting from Bed to Stretcher	Able to Perform	Able to Perform with Assistance	Unable to Perform	Initials/Date
15. Empty all drainage bags (e.g., T-tube, Hemo Vac, Jackson-Pratt). Record amounts. Secure drainage system to client's gown before transfer. *Comments:*	☐	☐	☐	
16. Move client to edge of bed near stretcher. Lift client up and over to avoid dragging. *Comments:*	☐	☐	☐	
17. Because client is now on side of bed with side rail down, the nurse on nonstretcher side of bed holds stretcher side of lift sheet up (by reaching across the client's chest) to prevent client from falling onto stretcher or off bed. *Comments:*	☐	☐	☐	
18. Place pillow or slider board to overlap bed and stretcher. *Comments:*	☐	☐	☐	
19. Have staff members grasp edges of lift sheet. Be sure to use good body mechanics. *Comments:*	☐	☐	☐	
20. On count of 3, have staff members pull lift sheet and client onto stretcher. *Comments:*	☐	☐	☐	
21. Position client on stretcher, place pillow under head, and cover with a sheet. *Comments:*	☐	☐	☐	

continued on the following page

continued from the previous page

Procedure 36-6 Assisting from Bed to Stretcher	Able to Perform	Able to Perform with Assistance	Unable to Perform	Initials/Date
22. Secure safety belts and elevate side rails of stretcher. *Comments:*	☐	☐	☐	
23. If IV pole is present, move it from bed IV pole to stretcher IV pole after client transfer. *Comments:*	☐	☐	☐	
24. Wash hands/hand hygiene. *Comments:*	☐	☐	☐	

Checklist for Procedure 36-7 Using a Hydraulic Lift

Name _____ Date _____

School _____

Instructor _____

Course _____

Procedure 36-7 Using a Hydraulic Lift	Able to Perform	Able to Perform with Assistance	Unable to Perform	Initials/Date
1. Wash hands/hand hygiene. *Comments:*	☐	☐	☐	
2. Check the health care provider's order to determine the time client may sit. *Comments:*	☐	☐	☐	
3. Check the client's medical history. *Comments:*	☐	☐	☐	
4. Ask client when last sat. *Comments:*	☐	☐	☐	
5. Lock wheels of bed. *Comments:*	☐	☐	☐	
6. Position chair close to bed. *Comments:*	☐	☐	☐	
7. Position urine drainage and NG and IV tubing on side of bed where chair will be placed. Ensure slack in tubing. *Comments:*	☐	☐	☐	
8. Clamp and disconnect any tubing. if permitted. *Comments:*	☐	☐	☐	

continued on the following page

continued from the previous page

Procedure 36-7 Using a Hydraulic Lift	Able to Perform	Able to Perform with Assistance	Unable to Perform	Initials/Date
9. Roll client on side and place sling on bed behind client. *Comments:*	☐	☐	☐	
10. Roll client on opposite side, then pull sling through and position it smoothly on bed. *Comments:*	☐	☐	☐	
11. Roll client back onto sling and fold arms over chest. *Comments:*	☐	☐	☐	
12. Make sure sling is centered. *Comments:*	☐	☐	☐	
13. Lower side rail and position lift on side of bed with chair. Spread base of hydraulic lift, as indicated in manufacturer's instructions, to provide stability. Protect from falls while side rail is down. *Comments:*	☐	☐	☐	
14. Lift frame and pass over client. Carefully lower frame and attach hooks to sling. *Comments:*	☐	☐	☐	
15. Raise client from bed by pumping handle. *Comments:*	☐	☐	☐	
16. Secure client with safety belt and cover client with blanket. *Comments:*	☐	☐	☐	

continued on the following page

continued from the previous page

Procedure 36-7 **Using a Hydraulic Lift**	**Able to Perform**	**Able to Perform with Assistance**	**Unable to Perform**	**Initials/Date**
17. Steer client away from bed and slide chair through base of lift. *Comments:*	☐	☐	☐	
18. The sling can be disconnected and lift can be moved out of way while client is sitting. If lift to be used to return client to bed, sling can be left in place beneath client. *Comments:*	☐	☐	☐	
19. Reposition and reconnect any tubing necessary. *Comments:*	☐	☐	☐	
20. Assess how client tolerated moving and sitting. *Comments:*	☐	☐	☐	
21. Place call light, appropriate covers, and padding, as needed after transfer. Place protective restraints, as needed. Cover feet with slippers if in sitting position. *Comments:*	☐	☐	☐	
22. Reverse the procedure to return client to bed. *Comments:*	☐	☐	☐	
23. Wash hands/hand hygiene. *Comments:*	☐	☐	☐	

Checklist for Procedure 36-8   Assisting with Ambulation and Safe Walking

Name _____ Date _____

School _____

Instructor _____

Course _____

Procedure 36-8 Assisting with Ambulation and Safe Walking	Able to Perform	Able to Perform with Assistance	Unable to Perform	Initials/Date
Ambulation Safety 1. Ambulating with IV: • Place IV pole with wheels at head of bed before having client dangle legs. • If possible, place a saline lock on IV. *Comments:*	☐	☐	☐	
2. Transfer IV from bed IV pole to portable IV pole. Client or nurse can guide portable IV pole during ambulation. *Comments:*	☐	☐	☐	
3. Ambulating with urinary drainage bags: • Empty bag before ambulation. • Have client sit on side of bed with legs dangling. • Remove urinary drainage bag from bed. • The nurse or client can hold the urinary drainage bag during ambulation. • Make sure drainage bag remains below level of bladder. *Comments:*	☐	☐	☐	
4. Ambulating with drainage tubes: • Secure tube and bag before ambulation. • Place rubber band around drainage tube near drainage bag. • Secure drainage tube and bag with safety pin through rubber band. • Allow slack. • The safety pin can be secured to client's gown or robe. *Comments:*	☐	☐	☐	

continued on the following page

continued from the previous page

Procedure 36-8 Assisting with Ambulation and Safe Walking	Able to Perform	Able to Perform with Assistance	Unable to Perform	Initials/Date
5. Ambulating with a chest tube drainage system: • Often requires two nurses, one assisting client and one nurse managing closed chest tube drainage system. • While client is sitting on edge of bed with feet dangling, remove hangers from drainage system. • Hold closed chest tube drainage system upright at all times to maintain water seal. • Do not pull or tug on chest tubes, because they may not be sutured into place. *Comments:*	☐	☐	☐	
6. Ambulating a client who is weak: • Use a transfer belt or gait belt. • For additional safety, a wheelchair can be pushed alongside client for ready access if client feels tired or faint. *Comments:*	☐	☐	☐	
7. If a client feels faint or dizzy during dangling, return client to supine position in bed and lower head of bed. Monitor client's blood pressure and pulse. *Comments:*	☐	☐	☐	
8. If client feels faint or dizzy during ambulation, allow client to sit in chair. Stay with client for safety. Request another nurse to secure a wheelchair, if not already available, to return client to bed. *Comments:*	☐	☐	☐	

continued on the following page

continued from the previous page

Procedure 36-8 **Assisting with Ambulation and Safe Walking**	**Able to Perform**	**Able to Perform with Assistance**	**Unable to Perform**	**Initials/Date**
9. If the client feels faint or dizzy during the ambulation and starts to fall, ease client to floor while supporting and protecting client's head. Position yourself next to and slightly behind the ambulating client to be able to step behind the client and safely ease the client to the floor. Ask other personnel to assist you in returning client to bed. Assess orthostatic blood pressures. *Comments:*	☐	☐	☐	
10. Encourage client to void before ambulating, especially if elderly. *Comments:*	☐	☐	☐	
Safe Walking 1. Hand hygiene. Inform client of the purposes and distance of the walking exercise. *Comments:*	☐	☐	☐	
2. Elevate the head of the bed and wait several minutes. *Comments:*	☐	☐	☐	
3. Lower the bed height. *Comments:*	☐	☐	☐	
4. With one arm on the client's back and one arm under the client's upper legs, move the client into position with legs dangling. *Comments:*	☐	☐	☐	
5. Encourage client to sit with legs dangling at side of bed for several minutes. *Comments:*	☐	☐	☐	

continued on the following page

continued from the previous page

Procedure 36-8 Assisting with Ambulation and Safe Walking	Able to Perform	Able to Perform with Assistance	Unable to Perform	Initials/Date
6. Place gait belt around client's waist and secure the buckle in front. *Comments:*	☐	☐	☐	
7. Stand in front of client with knees touching client's knees. *Comments:*	☐	☐	☐	
8. Place arms under client's axilla. *Comments:*	☐	☐	☐	
9. Assist client to a standing position, allowing client time to balance. *Comments:*	☐	☐	☐	
10. Help client ambulate the desired distance or distance of tolerance. Place your hand under client's forearm and ambulate close to client. Alternatively, place gait belt around client's waist and walk at client's side and slightly behind with one hand grasping the belt at center back. *Comments:*	☐	☐	☐	
11. Help client back to bed or chair. Make client comfortable, and make sure all lines and tubes are secure. *Comments:*	☐	☐	☐	
12. Wash hands/hand hygiene. *Comments:*	☐	☐	☐	

Checklist for Procedure 36-9   Assisting with Crutches, Cane, or Walker

Name _____ Date _____

School _____

Instructor _____

Course _____

Procedure 36-9 Assisting with Crutches, Cane, or Walker	Able to Perform	Able to Perform with Assistance	Unable to Perform	Initials/Date
Crutch Walking 1. Inform client that you will be assisting with ambulation using the device chosen. Wash hands/hand hygiene. *Comments:*	☐	☐	☐	
2. Assess client for strength, mobility, ROM, visual acuity, perceptual difficulties, and balance. *Comments:*	☐	☐	☐	
3. Measure client for size of crutches and adjust crutches to fit. While supine, measure client from heel to axilla. *Comments:*	☐	☐	☐	
4. Provide a robe or other covering as well as nonslip foot coverings or shoes. *Comments:*	☐	☐	☐	
5. Lower the height of the bed. *Comments:*	☐	☐	☐	
6. Have client at sit at side of bed with legs dangline for several minutes. Assess for vertigo or nausea. *Comments:*	☐	☐	☐	

continued on the following page

continued from the previous page

Procedure 36-9 Assisting with Crutches, Cane, or Walker	Able to Perform	Able to Perform with Assistance	Unable to Perform	Initials/Date
7. Apply gait belt around client's waist if balance and stability are unknown or unreliable. Good practice requires the use of a gait belt the first time client is out of bed. *Comments:*	☐	☐	☐	
8. Holding crutches: • Instruct client on method of holding crutches while client remains seated. • Elbows bent 30° while hands are on handgrips and pads 1.5 to 2 inches below axilla. • Instruct client to position crutches 4 to 5 inches laterally and 4 to 6 inches in front of feet. • Demonstrate this skill on yourself to increase client understanding. *Comments:*	☐	☐	☐	
9. Ambulating with crutches: • Assist client to standing position by placing both crutches in nondominant hand. • Have client use dominant hand to push off from bed while using crutches for balance. • Once erect, extra crutch can be moved into dominant hand. *Comments:*	☐	☐	☐	
10. Ambulating with crutches: • Instruct client to remain still for a few seconds while assessing for vertigo or nausea. • Stand close to client to support, as needed. • While client remains standing, check for correct fit of crutches. *Comments:*	☐	☐	☐	

continued on the following page

continued from the previous page

Procedure 36-9 Assisting with Crutches, Cane, or Walker	Able to Perform	Able to Perform with Assistance	Unable to Perform	Initials/Date
Four-Point Gait 11. Position crutches 4.5 to 6 inches to side and in front of each foot. Move right crutch forward 4 to 6 inches and move left foot forward, even with left crutch. Move left crutch forward 4 to 6 inches and move right foot forward, even with right crutch. Repeat four-point gait. *Comments:*	☐	☐	☐	
Three-Point Gait 12. Advance both crutches and the weaker leg forward together 4 to 6 inches. Move the stronger leg forward, even with the crutches. Repeat the three-point gate. *Comments:*	☐	☐	☐	
Two-Point Gait 13. Move the left crutch and right leg forward 4 to 6 inches. Move the right crutch and left leg forward 4 to 6 inches. Repeat the two-point gait. *Comments:*	☐	☐	☐	
Swing-Through Gait 14. This step is basically the same as the three-point gait. The difference is on the swing, whichever leg is moving will go past the stationary point and set down in front. *Comments:*	☐	☐	☐	
15. Walking Upstairs • Stand beside and slightly behind client. • Instruct client to position the crutches as if walking. • Place body weight on hands. Place the strong leg on the first step.	☐	☐	☐	

continued on the following page

continued from the previous page

Procedure 36-9 Assisting with Crutches, Cane, or Walker	Able to Perform	Able to Perform with Assistance	Unable to Perform	Initials/Date
• Pull the weak leg up and move the crutches up to the first step. • Repeat for all steps. *Comments:*				
16. Walking Downstairs • Position crutches as if walking. • Place weight on strong leg. • Move crutches down to next lower step. • Place partial weight on hands and crutches. • Move weak leg down to step with crutches. • Put total weight on arms and crutches. • Move strong leg to same step as weak leg and crutches. • Repeat for all steps. • A second caregiver standing behind client holding on to gait belt will further decrease risk of falling. *Comments:*	☐	☐	☐	
17. Set realistic goals and opportunities for progressive ambulation using crutches. *Comments:*	☐	☐	☐	
18. Consult with a physical therapist for clients learning to walk with crutches. *Comments:*	☐	☐	☐	
19. Wash hands/hand hygiene. *Comments:*	☐	☐	☐	
Sitting with Crutches 20. Instruct client to back up to chair until chair is felt with back of legs. *Comments:*	☐	☐	☐	

continued on the following page

continued from the previous page

Procedure 36-9 Assisting with Crutches, Cane, or Walker	Able to Perform	Able to Perform with Assistance	Unable to Perform	Initials/Date
21. Place both crutches in nondominant hand and have client use dominant hand to reach back to chair. *Comments:*	☐	☐	☐	
22. Instruct client to lower slowly into chair. *Comments:*	☐	☐	☐	
Walking with a Cane 23. Repeat 1–7. *Comments:*	☐	☐	☐	
24. Have client hold cane in hand opposite affected leg. Explain safety and body mechanics underlying use of a cane on the strong side. *Comments:*	☐	☐	☐	
25. Have client push up from sitting position while pushing down on bed with arms. *Comments:*	☐	☐	☐	
26. Have client stand at bedside for few moments. *Comments:*	☐	☐	☐	
27. Assess height of cane. With cane placed 6 inches ahead of client's body, top of cane should be at wrist level with the arm bent 25% to 30% at the elbow. *Comments:*	☐	☐	☐	

continued on the following page

continued from the previous page

Procedure 36-9 Assisting with Crutches, Cane, or Walker	Able to Perform	Able to Perform with Assistance	Unable to Perform	Initials/Date
28. Walk to side and slightly behind client, holding gait belt, if needed, for stability. *Comments:*	☐	☐	☐	
The Cane Gait 29. Have client move cane and weaker leg forward at same time for same distance. Have client place weight on weaker leg and cane, move the strong leg forward, and place weight on the strong leg. *Comments:*	☐	☐	☐	
Sitting with a Cane 30. Have client turn around and back up to chair. Have client grasp arm of chair with free hand and lower self into chair. Be sure to place cane out of way but within reach. *Comments:*	☐	☐	☐	
31. Set realistic goals and opportunities for progressive ambulation using a cane. *Comments:*	☐	☐	☐	
32. Consult with a physical therapist for clients learning to walk with a cane. *Comments:*	☐	☐	☐	
33. Wash hands/hand hygiene. *Comments:*	☐	☐	☐	
Walking with a Walker 34. Repeat 1–7. *Comments:*	☐	☐	☐	

continued on the following page

continued from the previous page

Procedure 36-9 Assisting with Crutches, Cane, or Walker	Able to Perform	Able to Perform with Assistance	Unable to Perform	Initials/Date
35. Place walker in front of client. *Comments:*	☐	☐	☐	
36. Have client put nondominant hand on front bar of walker or on handgrip for nondominant hand, whichever is more comfortable. Then, with client using dominant hand to push off from bed and nondominant hand for stabilization, help client to an erect position. *Comments:*	☐	☐	☐	
37. Have client transfer hand to the walker handgrips. *Comments:*	☐	☐	☐	
38. Be sure the walker is adjusted so the handgrips are just below waist level and client's arms are slightly bent at elbow. *Comments:*	☐	☐	☐	
39. Walk to side and slightly behind client, holding gait belt, if needed, for stability. *Comments:*	☐	☐	☐	
Walker Gait 40. Have client move the walker and the weaker leg forward at the same time (see Figure 36-76). Have client place as much weight as possible or walk as slowed on the weaker leg using the arms for supporting the rest of the weight. Have client move the strong leg forward and shift the weight to the strong leg (see Figure 36-77). *Comments:*	☐	☐	☐	

continued on the following page

continued from the previous page

Procedure 36-9 Assisting with Crutches, Cane, or Walker	Able to Perform	Able to Perform with Assistance	Unable to Perform	Initials/Date
Sitting with a Walker 41. Have the client turn around in front of the chair and back up until the back of the legs touch the chair. Have client place hands on the chair armrests, one hand at a time, then lower self into the chair using the armrests for support. *Comments:*	☐	☐	☐	

Checklist for Procedure 37-1   Obtaining a Wound Drainage Specimen for Culturing

Name _____ Date _____

School _____

Instructor _____

Course _____

Procedure 37-1 Obtaining a Wound Drainage Specimen for Culturing	Able to Perform	Able to Perform with Assistance	Unable to Perform	Initials/Date
1. Wash hands/hand hygiene. Apply disposable gloves. Remove old dressing. Place in moisture proof container and remove and discard gloves. Wash hands/ hand hygiene again. *Comments:*	☐	☐	☐	
2. Open dressing supplies using sterile technique and apply gloves. *Comments:*	☐	☐	☐	
3. Assess wound's appearance; note quality, quantity, color, and odor of discharge. *Comments:*	☐	☐	☐	
4. Irrigate wound with normal saline prior to culturing; do not irrigate with antiseptic. *Comments:*	☐	☐	☐	
5. Using a sterile gauze pad, absorb the excess saline, discard pad. *Comments:*	☐	☐	☐	
6. Remove culture tube from packaging. Remove culture swab from culture tube and gently roll swab over granulation tissue. Avoid eschar and wound edges. *Comments:*	☐	☐	☐	

continued on the following page

continued from the previous page

Procedure 37-1 Obtaining a Wound Drainage Specimen for Culturing	Able to Perform	Able to Perform with Assistance	Unable to Perform	Initials/Date
7. Replace swab into culture tube, being careful not to touch the swab to outside of tube. Recap tube. Crush ampule of medium located in bottom or cap of tube. *Comments:*	☐	☐	☐	
8. Remove gloves, wash hands/hand hygiene, and apply sterile gloves. Dress wound with sterile dressing. *Comments:*	☐	☐	☐	
9. Label specimen, place in biohazard transport bag, and arrange to transport specimen to laboratory, according to institutional policy. *Comments:*	☐	☐	☐	
10. Remove gloves. Wash hands/hand hygiene. *Comments:*	☐	☐	☐	
11. Document all assessment findings and actions taken. Document that a specimen was obtained. *Comments:*	☐	☐	☐	

Checklist for Procedure 37-2   Irrigating a Wound

Name _____ Date _____

School _____

Instructor _____

Course _____

Procedure 37-2 Irrigating a Wound	Able to Perform	Able to Perform with Assistance	Unable to Perform	Initials/Date
1. Confirm the health care practitioner's order. Note type and strength of ordered irrigation solution. *Comments:*	☐	☐	☐	
2. Assess client's pain level and medicate, if needed, with analgesic 30 minutes before procedure if po or IM pain medication. *Comments:*	☐	☐	☐	
3. Explain procedure to client. Wash hands/hand hygiene. *Comments:*	☐	☐	☐	
4. Place waterproof pad on bed. Assist client onto pad and into a position to allow irrigant to flow through wound and into basin from cleanest to dirtiest area of wound. *Comments:*	☐	☐	☐	
5. Wash hands/hand hygiene. Apply disposable gloves. Remove and discard old dressing. *Comments:*	☐	☐	☐	
6. Assess wound's appearance and note quality, quantity, color, and odor of drainage. *Comments:*	☐	☐	☐	

continued on the following page

continued from the previous page

Procedure 37-2 Irrigating a Wound	Able to Perform	Able to Perform with Assistance	Unable to Perform	Initials/Date
7. Remove and discard disposable gloves. Wash hands/hand hygiene. *Comments:*	☐	☐	☐	
8. Prepare sterile irrigation tray and dressing supplies. Pour room-temperature irrigation solution into solution container. *Comments:*	☐	☐	☐	
9. Apply sterile gloves (and goggles, if needed). *Comments:*	☐	☐	☐	
10. Position sterile basin below wound so irrigant will flow from cleanest area to dirtiest area and into basin. *Comments:*	☐	☐	☐	
11. Fill piston or bulb syringe with irrigant and gently flush wound. Hold syringe approximately 1 inch above wound bed to irrigate. Refill syringe and continue to flush wound until solution returns clear and no exudates is noted or until prescribed amount of fluid has been used. *Comments:*	☐	☐	☐	
12. Dry edges of wound with sterile gauze. *Comments:*	☐	☐	☐	
13. Assess wound's appearance and drainage. *Comments:*	☐	☐	☐	

continued on the following page

continued from the previous page

Procedure 37-2 Irrigating a Wound	Able to Perform	Able to Perform with Assistance	Unable to Perform	Initials/Date
14. Apply sterile dressing. Remove sterile gloves and dispose of properly. Wash hands/hand hygiene. *Comments:*	☐	☐	☐	
15. Document all assessment findings and actions taken. *Comments:*	☐	☐	☐	

Checklist for Procedure 37-3   Applying a Dry Dressing

Name _____ Date _____

School _____

Instructor _____

Course _____

Procedure 37-3 Applying a Dry Dressing	Able to Perform	Able to Perform with Assistance	Unable to Perform	Initials/Date
1. Gather supplies. *Comments:*	☐	☐	☐	
2. Provide privacy; draw curtains; close door. *Comments:*	☐	☐	☐	
3. Explain procedure to client. *Comments:*	☐	☐	☐	
4. Wash hands/hand hygiene. *Comments:*	☐	☐	☐	
5. Apply clean exam gloves. *Comments:*	☐	☐	☐	
6. Remove dressing and place in biohazard bag. Remove soiled gloves with contaminated surfaces inward and discard; apply clean gloves. *Comments:*	☐	☐	☐	
7. Assess appearance of wound bed for healing. *Comments:*	☐	☐	☐	

continued on the following page

continued from the previous page

Procedure 37-3 Applying a Dry Dressing	Able to Perform	Able to Perform with Assistance	Unable to Perform	Initials/Date
8. Cleanse skin around incision, if necessary, with a clean, warm, wet, washcloth. • If suture line requires cleansing, do gently. Use normal saline, half-strength hydrogen peroxide, or Betadine swab (consult orders of health care provider and/or institution policy) and cotton-tip applicators using a rolling motion. • Used applicators should not be reintroduced into sterile solution. *Comments:*	☐	☐	☐	
9. Remove used exam gloves. *Comments:*	☐	☐	☐	
10. Wash hands/hand hygiene. *Comments:*	☐	☐	☐	
11. Set up supplies. *Comments:*	☐	☐	☐	
12. Apply a new pair of clean exam gloves. *Comments:*	☐	☐	☐	
13. Grasping edges, apply a new dressing using 4 × 4 gauze pads folded to size 2 × 4. Place folded gauze pad lengthwise on wound and tape lightly or apply tubular mesh to patients with sensitive skin. Initial dressing; cite date and time was changed. *Comments:*	☐	☐	☐	

continued on the following page

continued from the previous page

Procedure 37-3 Applying a Dry Dressing	Able to Perform	Able to Perform with Assistance	Unable to Perform	Initials/Date
14. Remove gloves and dispose of appropriately. Wash hands/hand hygiene. *Comments:*	☐	☐	☐	
15. Conduct client and family session about the dressing, including teaching the dressing technique to the client and family. *Comments:*	☐	☐	☐	

Checklist for Procedure 37-4   Applying a Wet to Damp Dressing (Wet to Moist Dressing)

Name _____ Date _____

School _____

Instructor _____

Course _____

Procedure 37-4 Applying a Wet to Damp Dressing (Wet to Moist Dressing)	Able to Perform	Able to Perform with Assistance	Unable to Perform	Initials/Date
1. Review order of health care practitioner for wound care. Gather supplies. *Comments:*	☐	☐	☐	
2. Provide privacy; draw curtains; close door. *Comments:*	☐	☐	☐	
3. Assess need for pain medication. Assess need based on quality, pain pattern, location, and last pain medication received. *Comments:*	☐	☐	☐	
4. Explain procedure to client. *Comments:*	☐	☐	☐	
5. Wash hands/hand hygiene. *Comments:*	☐	☐	☐	
6. Apply clean exam gloves, a moisture-proof gown, mask, and eye protection, as appropriate. *Comments:*	☐	☐	☐	
7. Inform client that the dressing is going to be removed. *Comments:*	☐	☐	☐	

continued on the following page

continued from the previous page

Procedure 37-4 Applying a Wet to Damp Dressing (Wet to Moist Dressing)	Able to Perform	Able to Perform with Assistance	Unable to Perform	Initials/Date
8. Remove wet to damp dressing, noting number of gauze pads used, and place in appropriate receptacle. *Comments:*	☐	☐	☐	
9. Observe the undressed wound for healing (granulation and approximation of edges), signs of infection (inflammation, edema, warmth, pain), and drainage. *Comments:*	☐	☐	☐	
10. Cleanse skin around incision, if necessary, with a clean, warm, wet washcloth. *Comments:*	☐	☐	☐	
11. Remove used exam gloves. *Comments:*	☐	☐	☐	
12. Wash hands/hand hygiene. *Comments:*	☐	☐	☐	
13. Set up supplies in a sterile field, including pouring ordered solutions into appropriate containers, if indicated for dressing change. *Comments:*	☐	☐	☐	
14. Apply sterile gloves. *Comments:*	☐	☐	☐	

continued on the following page

continued from the previous page

Procedure 37-4 **Applying a Wet to Damp Dressing (Wet to Moist Dressing)**	**Able to Perform**	**Able to Perform with Assistance**	**Unable to Perform**	**Initials/Date**
15. Place gauze or packing material to be moistened in the bowl with the normal saline or other solution. • Wring gauze or packing of saline until damp. • Gently place damp gauze over the area. *Comments:*	☐	☐	☐	
16. Apply external dressing of dry 4 × 4 gauze pads, cover sponges, fluffs, or ABD pads. • Secure dressing in place with tape, Montgomery straps, or tubular mesh, as shown. *Comments:*	☐	☐	☐	
17. Remove glovesand wash hands/hand hygiene. *Comments:*	☐	☐	☐	
18. Mark dressing with date and time changed and initial it. *Comments:*	☐	☐	☐	
19. Conduct client and family education session about the dressing, which can include teaching the dressing technique to the client and family. *Comments:*	☐	☐	☐	

Checklist for Procedure 37-5   Preventing and Managing the Pressure Ulcer

Name _____ Date _____

School _____

Instructor _____

Course _____

Procedure 37-5 Preventing and Managing the Pressure Ulcer	Able to Perform	Able to Perform with Assistance	Unable to Perform	Initials/Date
1. Check health care practitioner's orders. *Comments:*	☐	☐	☐	
2. Gather equipment. *Comments:*	☐	☐	☐	
3. Identify client. Explain procedure. *Comments:*	☐	☐	☐	
4. Wash hands/hand hygiene. *Comments:*	☐	☐	☐	
5. Provide privacy. Apply gloves. *Comments:*	☐	☐	☐	
6. Adjust bed to your level and lower side rail nearest you without leaving client unattended. *Comments:*	☐	☐	☐	
7. Assess client's risk for pressure ulcers by using the Braden scale or a similar chart. *Comments:*	☐	☐	☐	
8. Assess client's skin over all pressure points *Comments:*	☐	☐	☐	

continued on the following page

continued from the previous page

Procedure 37-5 Preventing and Managing the Pressure Ulcer	Able to Perform	Able to Perform with Assistance	Unable to Perform	Initials/Date
9. Assess other sites for potential areas of pressure. *Comments:*	☐	☐	☐	
10. Change client's position. *Comments:*	☐	☐	☐	
11. Keep client's position at 30° angle or less. *Comments:*	☐	☐	☐	
12. Provide skin care if area is soiled or sweaty, but do not massage pressure points. *Comments:*	☐	☐	☐	
13. Use support devices to support the body. *Comments:*	☐	☐	☐	
14. Perform dressing change to a pressure ulcer, as ordered or per agency policy. *Comments:*	☐	☐	☐	
15. Return side rail to upright position and lower bed. *Comments:*	☐	☐	☐	
16. Remove gloves. Wash hands/hand hygiene. *Comments:*	☐	☐	☐	

continued on the following page

continued from the previous page

Procedure 37-5 **Preventing and Managing the Pressure Ulcer**	**Able to Perform**	**Able to Perform with Assistance**	**Unable to Perform**	**Initials/Date**
17. Document appearance of pressure points and/or ulcers, skin care, wound care provided, and position changes. *Comments:*	☐	☐	☐	
18. Create an every-2-hour turning schedule, if one is not available. *Comments:*	☐	☐	☐	

Checklist for Procedure 39-1   Assisting with a Bedpan or Urinal

Name _____ Date _____

School _____

Instructor _____

Course _____

Procedure 39-1 Assisting with a Bedpan or Urinal	Able to Perform	Able to Perform with Assistance	Unable to Perform	Initials/Date
Positioning a Bedpan 1. Close curtain or door. *Comments:*	☐	☐	☐	
2. Wash hands/hand hygiene; apply gloves. *Comments:*	☐	☐	☐	
3. Lower head of bed. *Comments:*	☐	☐	☐	
4. Elevate bed. *Comments:*	☐	☐	☐	
5. Assist client to side-lying position using side rail for support. *Comments:*	☐	☐	☐	
6. Place bedpan under buttocks. Place a fracture pan with lower end near client's lower back region. Place large bedpans with opening near client's thighs. *Comments:*	☐	☐	☐	
7. While holding bedpan with one hand, help client roll onto back, while pushing against bedpan (toward center of bed) to hold in place. *Comments:*	☐	☐	☐	

continued on the following page

continued from the previous page

Procedure 39-1 Assisting with a Bedpan or Urinal	Able to Perform	Able to Perform with Assistance	Unable to Perform	Initials/Date
8. Alternate: Help client raise hips using overbed trapeze and slide pan in place. Alternate: If client is unable to turn or raise hips, use a fracture pan instead of a bedpan. With fracture pan, flat side is placed toward client's head. *Comments:*	☐	☐	☐	
9. Check placement of bedpan between client's legs. *Comments:*	☐	☐	☐	
10. If indicated, elevate head of bed to 45° angle or higher, for comfort. *Comments:*	☐	☐	☐	
11. Place call light within reach of client, place side rails in upright position, lower bed, and provide privacy. *Comments:*	☐	☐	☐	
12. Remove gloves; wash hands/hand hygiene. *Comments:*	☐	☐	☐	
Positioning a Urinal 13. Repeat Actions 1 and 2. *Comments:*	☐	☐	☐	
14. Lift covers and place urinal so client can grasp handle and position it. If client cannot do this, you must position urinal and place penis into opening. *Comments:*	☐	☐	☐	

continued on the following page

continued from the previous page

Procedure 39-1 Assisting with a Bedpan or Urinal	Able to Perform	Able to Perform with Assistance	Unable to Perform	Initials/Date
15. Remove gloves; wash hands/hand hygiene. *Comments:*	☐	☐	☐	
Removing a Bedpan 16. Wash hands/hand hygiene; apply gloves. *Comments:*	☐	☐	☐	
17. Gather toilet paper and washing supplies. *Comments:*	☐	☐	☐	
18. Lower head of bed to supine position. *Comments:*	☐	☐	☐	
19. While holding bedpan with one hand, roll client to side and remove pan, being careful not to pull or shear skin sticking to pan or to spill contents. *Comments:*	☐	☐	☐	
20. Assist with cleaning or wiping; always wipe with front to back motion. *Comments:*	☐	☐	☐	
21. Empty bedpan (observe and measure urine output and check for occult blood, if ordered), clean bedpan, and store in proper place; if bedpan is emptied outside client's room, cover during transport. *Comments:*	☐	☐	☐	
22. Remove soiled gloves. Wash hands/hand hygiene. *Comments:*	☐	☐	☐	

continued on the following page

continued from the previous page

Procedure 39-1 Assisting with a Bedpan or Urinal	Able to Perform	Able to Perform with Assistance	Unable to Perform	Initials/Date
23. Allow client to wash hands. *Comments:*	☐	☐	☐	
24. Place call light within reach; recheck that side rails are in upright position. *Comments:*	☐	☐	☐	
25. Wash hands/hand hygiene. *Comments:*	☐	☐	☐	
Removing a Urinal 26. Hand hygiene and apply gloves. *Comments:*	☐	☐	☐	
27. Empty urinal, measuring urine output if ordered; rinse urinal and replace within client's reach. Observe odor and color of urine before discarding. *Comments:*	☐	☐	☐	
28. Remove soiled gloves; wash hands. *Comments:*	☐	☐	☐	
29. Allow client to wash hands. *Comments:*	☐	☐	☐	
30. Place call light within reach; recheck that side rails are in upright position. *Comments:*	☐	☐	☐	
31. Wash hands/hand hygiene. *Comments:*	☐	☐	☐	

Checklist for Procedure 39-2   Applying a Condom Catheter

Name _____ Date _____

School _____

Instructor _____

Course _____

Procedure 39-2 Applying a Condom Catheter	Able to Perform	Able to Perform with Assistance	Unable to Perform	Initials/Date
1. Wash hands/hand hygiene. *Comments:*	☐	☐	☐	
2. Protect client's privacy by closing door and pulling curtains around bed. *Comments:*	☐	☐	☐	
3. Position client in comfortable position, preferably supine, if tolerated. Raise bed to a comfortable height for nurse. *Comments:*	☐	☐	☐	
4. Apply latex-free gloves. *Comments:*	☐	☐	☐	
5. Fold client's gown across abdomen and pull sheet up over client's legs. *Comments:*	☐	☐	☐	
6. Assess client's penis for any signs of redness, irritation, or skin breakdown. *Comments:*	☐	☐	☐	
7. Clean client's penis with warm soapy water. Retract foreskin on uncircumcised male and clean thoroughly in folds. *Comments:*	☐	☐	☐	

continued on the following page

continued from the previous page

Procedure 39-2 Applying a Condom Catheter	Able to Perform	Able to Perform with Assistance	Unable to Perform	Initials/Date
8. Return client's foreskin to its normal position. *Comments:*	☐	☐	☐	
9. Shave any excess hair around base of penis, if required by institutional policy. *Comments:*	☐	☐	☐	
10. Rinse and dry area. *Comments:*	☐	☐	☐	
11. If condom kit is used, open package containing skin preparation. Wipe and apply skin preparation solution to penis shaft. If client has an erection, wait for termination of erection before applying catheter. *Comments:*	☐	☐	☐	
12. Apply double-sided adhesive strip around base of penis in spiral fashion, 1 inch from proximal end of penis. Do not completely encircle penis or tightly encompass penis. *Comments:*	☐	☐	☐	
13. Position rolled condom at distal portion of penis and unroll it, covering penis and double-sided strip of adhesive. Leave a 1- to 2-inch space between penis tip and condom end. *Comments:*	☐	☐	☐	
14. Gently press condom to adhesive strip. *Comments:*	☐	☐	☐	

continued on the following page

continued from the previous page

Procedure 39-2 Applying a Condom Catheter	Able to Perform	Able to Perform with Assistance	Unable to Perform	Initials/Date
15. Attach drainage bag tubing to catheter tubing. Make sure tubing lays over client's legs, not under. Secure drainage bag to side of bed below level of client's bladder or to client's leg. *Comments:*	☐	☐	☐	
16. Determine that condom and tubing are not twisted. *Comments:*	☐	☐	☐	
17. Cover client. *Comments:*	☐	☐	☐	
18. Dispose of used equipment in appropriate receptacle; wash hands/ hand hygiene. *Comments:*	☐	☐	☐	
19. Return bed to lowest position and reposition client to comfortable or appropriate position. *Comments:*	☐	☐	☐	
20. Empty bag, measure urinary output, and record every 4 hours. After procedure, remove gloves: wash hands/ hand hygiene. *Comments:*	☐	☐	☐	
21. Remove condom once a day to clean area and assess skin for signs of impaired skin integrity. *Comments:*	☐	☐	☐	

Checklist for Procedure 39-3   Inserting an Indwelling Catheter: Male

Name _____ Date _____

School _____

Instructor _____

Course _____

Procedure 39-3 Inserting an Indwelling Catheter: Male	Able to Perform	Able to Perform with Assistance	Unable to Perform	Initials/Date
Performing Urinary Catheterization: Male Client 1. Gather equipment and any supplies not in the prepackaged kit. Wash hands/ hand hygiene. *Comments:*	☐	☐	☐	
2. Provide for privacy and explain procedure to client. *Comments:*	☐	☐	☐	
3. Set bed to comfortable height to work and raise side rail on side opposite you. *Comments:*	☐	☐	☐	
4. Assist client to supine position with legs slightly spread. *Comments:*	☐	☐	☐	
5. Drape client's abdomen and thighs, if needed. *Comments:*	☐	☐	☐	
6. Ensure adequate lighting of penis and perineal area. *Comments:*	☐	☐	☐	
7. Wash hands/hand hygiene; apply latex-free disposable gloves; wash perineal area. *Comments:*	☐	☐	☐	

continued on the following page

continued from the previous page

Procedure 39-3 Inserting an Indwelling Catheter: Male	Able to Perform	Able to Perform with Assistance	Unable to Perform	Initials/Date
8. Remove gloves; wash hands/hand hygiene. *Comments:*	☐	☐	☐	
9. Open catheterization kit, using aseptic technique. Use wrapper to establish sterile field. *Comments:*	☐	☐	☐	
10. If catheter is not included in kit, carefully drop sterile catheter onto field using aseptic technique. Add any other items needed. *Comments:*	☐	☐	☐	
11. Apply sterile gloves. *Comments:*	☐	☐	☐	
12. Place fenestrated drape from catheterization kit over client's perineal area with penis extending through opening. *Comments:*	☐	☐	☐	
13. If inserting retention catheter, attach syringe filled with sterile water to Luer-Lok tail of catheter. Inflate and deflate retention balloon. Detach water-filled syringe. *Comments:*	☐	☐	☐	
14. Attach catheter to urine drainage bag, if not preconnected. *Comments:*	☐	☐	☐	

continued on the following page

continued from the previous page

Procedure 39-3 Inserting an Indwelling Catheter: Male	Able to Perform	Able to Perform with Assistance	Unable to Perform	Initials/Date
15. Generously coat distal portion of catheter with water-soluble, sterile lubricant and place nearby on sterile field. *Comments:*	☐	☐	☐	
16. With nondominant hand, gently grasp penis and retract foreskin (if present). With dominant hand, cleanse glans penis with povidone-iodine solution or other antimicrobial cleanser. *Comments:*	☐	☐	☐	
17. Hold penis perpendicular to body and pull up gently. *Comments:*	☐	☐	☐	
18. Insert 10 ml sterile, water-soluble lubricant (use a 2% Xylocaine lubricant, whenever feasible) into urethra. *Comments:*	☐	☐	☐	
19. Holding catheter in dominant hand, steadily insert catheter about 8 inches, until urine is noted in drainage bag or tubing. *Comments:*	☐	☐	☐	
20. If catheter will be removed as client's bladder is empty, insert catheter another inch, place penis in comfortable position, and hold catheter in place as bladder drains. *Comments:*	☐	☐	☐	

continued on the following page

continued from the previous page

Procedure 39-3 Inserting an Indwelling Catheter: Male	Able to Perform	Able to Perform with Assistance	Unable to Perform	Initials/Date
21. If catheter will be indwelling with retention balloon, continue inserting until hub of catheter (bifurcation between drainage port and retention balloon arm) is met. *Comments:*	☐	☐	☐	
22. Reattach water-filled syringe to inflation port. *Comments:*	☐	☐	☐	
23. Inflate retention balloon with sterile water, per manufacturer's recommendations or prescribing practitioner's orders. *Comments:*	☐	☐	☐	
24. Instruct client to immediately report discomfort or pressure during balloon inflation; if pain occurs, discontinue procedure, deflate balloon, and insert catheter farther into bladder. If client continues to complain of pain with balloon inflation, remove catheter and notify client's health care provider. *Comments:*	☐	☐	☐	
25. Once balloon is inflated, gently pull catheter until retention balloon rests snugly against bladder neck (resistance will be felt when balloon is properly seated). *Comments:*	☐	☐	☐	
26. Secure catheter according to institutional policy. Securing to either client's thigh or abdomen is generally acceptable. *Comments:*	☐	☐	☐	

continued on the following page

continued from the previous page

Procedure 39-3 Inserting an Indwelling Catheter: Male	Able to Perform	Able to Perform with Assistance	Unable to Perform	Initials/Date
27. Place drainage bag below level of bladder. Do not let rest on floor. Secure drainage tubing to prevent pulling on tubing and catheter. *Comments:*	☐	☐	☐	
28. Remove gloves, dispose of equipment. Wash hands/hand hygiene. *Comments:*	☐	☐	☐	
29. Help client adjust position. Lower bed. *Comments:*	☐	☐	☐	
30. Assess and document amount, color, odor, and quality of urine. *Comments:*	☐	☐	☐	

Checklist for Procedure 39-4   Inserting an Indwelling Catheter: Female

Name _____ Date _____

School _____

Instructor _____

Course _____

Procedure 39-4 Inserting an Indwelling Catheter: Female	Able to Perform	Able to Perform with Assistance	Unable to Perform	Initials/Date
Performing Urinary Catheterization 1. Gather equipment. Read label on catheterization kit. Gather supplies needed. *Comments:*	☐	☐	☐	
2. Provide for privacy and explain procedure to client. Assess for allergy to povidone-iodine. Wash hands/hand hygiene. *Comments:*	☐	☐	☐	
3. Set bed to comfortable height to work, and raise side rail on side opposite you. *Comments:*	☐	☐	☐	
4. Assist client to supine position with legs spread and feet together or to a side-lying position with upper leg flexed. *Comments:*	☐	☐	☐	
5. Drape client's abdomen and thighs for warmth, if needed. *Comments:*	☐	☐	☐	
6. Ensure adequate lighting of perineal area. *Comments:*	☐	☐	☐	

continued on the following page

continued from the previous page

Procedure 39-4 Inserting an Indwelling Catheter: Female	Able to Perform	Able to Perform with Assistance	Unable to Perform	Initials/Date
7. Wash hands/hand hygiene; apply disposable gloves. *Comments:*	☐	☐	☐	
8. Wash perineal area. *Comments:*	☐	☐	☐	
9. Remove gloves and wash hands. *Comments:*	☐	☐	☐	
10. Open catheterization kit, using aseptic technique. Use wrapper for sterile field. *Comments:*	☐	☐	☐	
11. If catheter is not included in kit, drop sterile catheter onto field using aseptic technique. Add any other items needed. *Comments:*	☐	☐	☐	
12. Apply sterile gloves. *Comments:*	☐	☐	☐	
13. If inserting a retention catheter, attach syringe filled with sterile water to Luer-Lok tail of catheter. Inflate and deflate retention balloon. Detach water-filled syringe. *Comments:*	☐	☐	☐	
14. Attach catheter to urine drainage bag if not preconnected. *Comments:*	☐	☐	☐	

continued on the following page

continued from the previous page

Procedure 39-4 Inserting an Indwelling Catheter: Female	Able to Perform	Able to Perform with Assistance	Unable to Perform	Initials/Date
15. Generously coat distal portion of catheter with water-soluble, sterile lubricant and place nearby on sterile field. *Comments:*	☐	☐	☐	
16. Place fenestrated drape from catheterization kit over client's perineal area with labia visible through opening. *Comments:*	☐	☐	☐	
17. Gently spread labia minora with fingers of nondominant hand and visualize urinary meatus. *Comments:*	☐	☐	☐	
18. Holding labia apart with nondominant hand, use forceps to pick up cotton ball soaked in povidone-iodine, and cleanse periurethral mucosa. Use one downward stroke for each cotton ball and dispose. Keep labia separated with nondominant hand until catheter inserted. *Comments:*	☐	☐	☐	
19. Holding catheter in dominant hand, steadily insert it into meatus until urine is noted in drainage bag or tubing. *Comments:*	☐	☐	☐	
20. If catheter will be removed as soon as client's bladder is empty, insert catheter another inch and hold catheter in place as bladder drains. *Comments:*	☐	☐	☐	

continued on the following page

continued from the previous page

Procedure 39-4 Inserting an Indwelling Catheter: Female	Able to Perform	Able to Perform with Assistance	Unable to Perform	Initials/Date
21. If catheter will be indwelling with retention balloon, continue inserting another 1–3 inches. *Comments:*	☐	☐	☐	
22. Reattach water-filled syringe to inflation port. *Comments:*	☐	☐	☐	
23. Inflate retention balloon using manufacturer's recommendations or according to prescribing practitioner's orders. *Comments:*	☐	☐	☐	
24. Instruct client to immediately report discomfort or pressure during balloon inflation; if pain occurs, discontinue procedure, deflate balloon, and insert catheter farther into bladder. If client continues to complain of pain with balloon inflation, remove catheter and notify client's health care provider. *Comments:*	☐	☐	☐	
25. Once balloon has been inflated, gently pull catheter until retention balloon is resting snugly against bladder neck (resistance will be felt when balloon is properly seated). *Comments:*	☐	☐	☐	
26. Tape catheter to abdomen or thigh snugly, with enough slack not to pull on bladder. *Comments:*	☐	☐	☐	

continued on the following page

continued from the previous page

Procedure 39-4 Inserting an Indwelling Catheter: Female	Able to Perform	Able to Perform with Assistance	Unable to Perform	Initials/Date
27. Place drainage bag below level of bladder. Do not let rest on floor. Make sure tubing lies over, not under, leg. *Comments:*	☐	☐	☐	
28. Remove gloves, dispose of equipment. Wash hands/hand hygiene. *Comments:*	☐	☐	☐	
29. Help client adjust position. Lower bed. *Comments:*	☐	☐	☐	
30. Assess and document amount, color, odor, and quality of urine. *Comments:*	☐	☐	☐	
31. Wash hands/hand hygiene. *Comments:*	☐	☐	☐	

Checklist for Procedure 39-5   Irrigating an Open Urinary Catheter

Name _____ Date _____

School _____

Instructor _____

Course _____

Procedure 39-5 Irrigating an Open Urinary Catheter	Able to Perform	Able to Perform with Assistance	Unable to Perform	Initials/Date
1. Verify need for bladder or catheter irrigation. *Comments:*	☐	☐	☐	
2. For prn catheter irrigation, palpate for full bladder and check current output against previous totals. *Comments:*	☐	☐	☐	
3. Verify prescribing practitioner's orders for type of irrigation and irrigant, as well as amount. *Comments:*	☐	☐	☐	
4. If repeat procedure, read previous documentation in record. *Comments:*	☐	☐	☐	
5. Assemble supplies. Wash hands/hand hygiene. *Comments:*	☐	☐	☐	
6. Premedicate client, if ordered or needed. *Comments:*	☐	☐	☐	
7. Provide teaching to client, as needed. *Comments:*	☐	☐	☐	

continued on the following page

continued from the previous page

Procedure 39-5 Irrigating an Open Urinary Catheter	Able to Perform	Able to Perform with Assistance	Unable to Perform	Initials/Date
8. Assist client to dorsal recumbent position. *Comments:*	☐	☐	☐	
9. Wash hands/hand hygiene. *Comments:*	☐	☐	☐	
10. Provide for client privacy with a closed door or curtain. *Comments:*	☐	☐	☐	
11. Empty urine collection bag. *Comments:*	☐	☐	☐	
12. Expose retention catheter and place water-resistant drape underneath it. *Comments:*	☐	☐	☐	
13. Open sterile syringe and container. Stand it up carefully in or on the wrapper and add 100–200 cc sterile diluent without touching or contaminating syrinte tip or inside of receptacle. *Comments:*	☐	☐	☐	
14. Open end of antiseptic swab package, exposing swab sticks. *Comments:*	☐	☐	☐	
15. Open sterile cover for drainage tube. *Comments:*	☐	☐	☐	
16. Apply sterile gloves. *Comments:*	☐	☐	☐	

continued on the following page

continued from the previous page

Procedure 39-5 Irrigating an Open Urinary Catheter	Able to Perform	Able to Perform with Assistance	Unable to Perform	Initials/Date
17. Disinfect connection between catheter and drainage tubing. *Comments:*	☐	☐	☐	
18. After disinfectant dries, loosen connection ends. *Comments:*	☐	☐	☐	
19. Grasp catheter and tubing 1–2 inches from ends, with catheter in nondominant hand. *Comments:*	☐	☐	☐	
20. Fold catheter to pinch it closed between palm and last three fingers, use thumb and first finger to hold sterile cap for drainage tube. *Comments:*	☐	☐	☐	
21. Separate catheter and tube, covering tube tightly with sterile cap. *Comments:*	☐	☐	☐	
22. Fill syringe with 30 cc for catheter irrigation, 60 cc for bladder irrigation. Insert tip of syringe into catheter and gently instill solution into catheter. *Comments:*	☐	☐	☐	
23. Clamp catheter, if ordered (medicated solution); if not, clamped irrigant may be released into a collection container or aspirated back into syringe. *Comments:*	☐	☐	☐	

continued on the following page

continued from the previous page

Procedure 39-5 Irrigating an Open Urinary Catheter	Able to Perform	Able to Perform with Assistance	Unable to Perform	Initials/Date
24. If bladder or catheter being irrigated to clear solid material, repeat irrigation until return clear. *Comments:*	☐	☐	☐	
25. Reconnect system and remove sterile gloves. Wash hands/hand hygiene. *Comments:*	☐	☐	☐	
26. When irrigation is finished, record type of returns and total amount of irrigation fluid used. *Comments:*	☐	☐	☐	
27. Monitor client for pain, urine color and clarity, any solid material passed, and total intake and output. *Comments:*	☐	☐	☐	
28. Wash hands/hand hygiene. *Comments:*	☐	☐	☐	

Checklist for Procedure 39-6   Irrigating the Bladder Using a Closed-System Catheter

Name _____ Date _____

School _____

Instructor _____

Course _____

Procedure 39-6 Irrigating the Bladder Using a Closed-System Catheter	Able to Perform	Able to Perform with Assistance	Unable to Perform	Initials/Date
Intermittent Bladder Irrigation Using a Standard Retention Catheter and a Y Adapter 1. Wash hands/hand hygiene. *Comments:*	☐	☐	☐	
2. Provide privacy. *Comments:*	☐	☐	☐	
3. Hang prescribed irrigation solution from IV pole. *Comments:*	☐	☐	☐	
4. Insert clamped irrigation tubing into bottle of irrigant and prime tubing with fluid, expelling air and reclamping tube. *Comments:*	☐	☐	☐	
5. Prepare sterile antiseptic swabs and sterile Y connector, if used. *Comments:*	☐	☐	☐	
6. Apply sterile gloves. *Comments:*	☐	☐	☐	
7. Clamp urinary catheter. *Comments:*	☐	☐	☐	
8. Unhook drainage bag from retention catheter. *Comments:*	☐	☐	☐	

continued on the following page

continued from the previous page

Procedure 39-6 **Irrigating the Bladder Using a Closed-System Catheter**	**Able to Perform**	**Able to Perform with Assistance**	**Unable to Perform**	**Initials/Date**
9. While holding drainage tubing and drainage port of catheter in nondominant hand, cleanse both tubing and port with antiseptic swabs. *Comments:*	☐	☐	☐	
10. Connect one port of Y connector to drainage port of retention catheter. *Comments:*	☐	☐	☐	
11. Connect another port of Y adapter to drainage tubing and bag. *Comments:*	☐	☐	☐	
12. Attach third port of Y adapter to irrigant tubing. *Comments:*	☐	☐	☐	
13. Unclamp urinary catheter and establish that urine is draining through catheter into drainage bag. *Comments:*	☐	☐	☐	
14. To irrigate catheter and bladder, clamp drainage tubing distal to Y adapter. *Comments:*	☐	☐	☐	
15. Instill prescribed amount of irrigant. *Comments:*	☐	☐	☐	
16. Clamp irrigant tubing. *Comments:*	☐	☐	☐	

continued on the following page

continued from the previous page

Procedure 39-6 Irrigating the Bladder Using a Closed-System Catheter	Able to Perform	Able to Perform with Assistance	Unable to Perform	Initials/Date
17. If prescribing practitioner has ordered irrigant to remain in bladder for a measured length of time, wait prescribed time. *Comments:*	☐	☐	☐	
18. Unclamp drainage tubing and monitor drainage as it flows into drainage bag. *Comments:*	☐	☐	☐	
Closed Bladder Irrigation Using a Three-Way Catheter 19. Wash hands/hand hygiene. *Comments:*	☐	☐	☐	
20. Provide privacy. *Comments:*	☐	☐	☐	
21. Explain procedure to client. Provide support. *Comments:*	☐	☐	☐	
22. Hang prescribed irrigation solution from IV pole. *Comments:*	☐	☐	☐	
23. Insert clamped irrigation tubing into bottle of irrigant and prime tubing with fluid, expelling air and reclamping tube. *Comments:*	☐	☐	☐	
24. Prepare sterile antiseptic swabs and any other sterile equipment needed. *Comments:*	☐	☐	☐	

continued on the following page

continued from the previous page

Procedure 39-6 Irrigating the Bladder Using a Closed-System Catheter	Able to Perform	Able to Perform with Assistance	Unable to Perform	Initials/Date
25. Apply sterile gloves. *Comments:*	☐	☐	☐	
26. Clamp urinary catheter. *Comments:*	☐	☐	☐	
27. Remove cap from irrigation port of three-way catheter. *Comments:*	☐	☐	☐	
28. Cleanse irrigation port with sterile antiseptic swabs. *Comments:*	☐	☐	☐	
29. Attach irrigation tubing to irrigation port of three-way catheter. *Comments:*	☐	☐	☐	
30. Remove clamp from catheter and observe for urine drainage. *Comments:*	☐	☐	☐	
If intermittent irrigation has been ordered: 31. Instill prescribed amount of irrigant. *Comments:*	☐	☐	☐	
32. Clamp irrigant tubing. *Comments:*	☐	☐	☐	
33. If prescribing practitioner has ordered irrigant to remain in bladder for a measured length of time, clamp drainage tube before instilling irrigant and wait prescribed length of time. *Comments:*	☐	☐	☐	

continued on the following page

continued from the previous page

Procedure 39-6 Irrigating the Bladder Using a Closed-System Catheter	Able to Perform	Able to Perform with Assistance	Unable to Perform	Initials/Date
34. Monitor drainage as flows into drainage bag. *Comments:*	☐	☐	☐	
35. Tape catheter securely to thigh. *Comments:*	☐	☐	☐	
36. Wash hands/hand hygiene. *Comments:*	☐	☐	☐	
If continuous bladder irrigation has been ordered: 37. Adjust clamp on irrigation tubing to allow prescribed rate of irrigant to flow into catheter and bladder. *Comments:*	☐	☐	☐	
38. Monitor drainage for color, clarity, debris, and volume as it flows into drainage bag. *Comments:*	☐	☐	☐	
39. Tape catheter securely to thigh. *Comments:*	☐	☐	☐	
40. Wash hands/hand hygiene. *Comments:*	☐	☐	☐	

Checklist for Procedure 39-7   Administering an Enema

Name _____ Date _____

School _____

Instructor _____

Course _____

Procedure 39-7 Administering an Enema	Able to Perform	Able to Perform with Assistance	Unable to Perform	Initials/Date
Large-Volume Cleansing Enema 1. Wash hands/hand hygiene. *Comments:*	☐	☐	☐	
2. Assess client's understanding of procedure and provide privacy. *Comments:*	☐	☐	☐	
3. Apply gloves. *Comments:*	☐	☐	☐	
4. Prepare equipment. *Comments:*	☐	☐	☐	
5. Place absorbent pad on bed under client. Assist client into left lateral position with right leg flexed. If needed, place a bedpan on bed nearby. *Comments:*	☐	☐	☐	
6. If specified, heat solution to desired temperature using thermometer to measure. *Comments:*	☐	☐	☐	
7. Pour solution into bag or bucket; add water, if needed. Open clamp and allow solution to prime tubing. Clamp tubing when primed. *Comments:*	☐	☐	☐	

continued on the following page

continued from the previous page

Procedure 39-7 Administering an Enema	Able to Perform	Able to Perform with Assistance	Unable to Perform	Initials/Date
8. Lubricate 5 cm (2 inches) of rectal tube unless it is prelubricated. *Comments:*	☐	☐	☐	
9. Holding enema container level with rectum, have client take deep breath. Slowly and smoothly insert rectal tube into rectum approximately 7–10 cm in an adult. Aim rectal tube toward client's umbilicus. *Comments:*	☐	☐	☐	
10. Raise container holding solution 12–18 inches for an adult and open clamp. Solution can be placed on IV pole at proper height. *Comments:*	☐	☐	☐	
11. Slowly administer fluid. *Comments:*	☐	☐	☐	
12. When solution completely administered or when client cannot hold any more fluid, clamp tubing; remove rectal tube and dispose properly. *Comments:*	☐	☐	☐	
13. Clean lubricant, solution, and any feces from anus with toilet tissue. *Comments:*	☐	☐	☐	
14. Have client continue to lie on left side for prescribed time. *Comments:*	☐	☐	☐	

continued on the following page

continued from the previous page

Procedure 39-7 Administering an Enema	Able to Perform	Able to Perform with Assistance	Unable to Perform	Initials/Date
15. When client has retained enema for prescribed time, assist to bedside commode, toilet, or onto bedpan. If client is using bathroom, instruct not to flush toilet when finished. *Comments:*	☐	☐	☐	
16. When client is finished expelling enema, assist to clean perineal area, if needed. *Comments:*	☐	☐	☐	
17. Return client to comfortable position. Place clean, dry protective pad under client to catch any solution or feces. *Comments:*	☐	☐	☐	
18. Observe feces and document data. *Comments:*	☐	☐	☐	
19. Remove gloves; wash hands/hand hygiene. *Comments:*	☐	☐	☐	
Small-Volume Prepackaged Enema 20. Wash hands/hand hygiene. *Comments:*	☐	☐	☐	
21. Remove enema from packaging. Review instructions. Packaged enema can be placed in basin of warm water to warm fluid before use. *Comments:*	☐	☐	☐	
22. Apply gloves. *Comments:*	☐	☐	☐	

continued on the following page

continued from the previous page

Procedure 39-7 Administering an Enema	Able to Perform	Able to Perform with Assistance	Unable to Perform	Initials/Date
23. Place absorbent pad on bed under client. Assist client into left lateral position with right leg flexed sharply or use knee-chest position. If needed, place a bedpan nearby. *Comments:*	☐	☐	☐	
24. Remove protective cap from nozzle and inspect nozzle for lubrication. If needed, add more. *Comments:*	☐	☐	☐	
25. Squeeze container gently to remove air and prime nozzle. *Comments:*	☐	☐	☐	
26. Have client take deep breath. Simultaneously, gently insert enema nozzle into anus, pointing nozzle toward umbilicus. *Comments:*	☐	☐	☐	
27. Squeeze container until all solution instilled. *Comments:*	☐	☐	☐	
28. Remove nozzle from anus and dispose of empty container. *Comments:*	☐	☐	☐	
29. Clean lubricant, solution, and any feces from anus with tissue. *Comments:*	☐	☐	☐	

continued on the following page

continued from the previous page

Procedure 39-7 Administering an Enema	Able to Perform	Able to Perform with Assistance	Unable to Perform	Initials/Date
30. Have client continue to lie on left side for prescribed time. *Comments:*	☐	☐	☐	
31. When client has retained enema for prescribed time, assist to bedside commode, toilet, or onto bedpan. If client using bathroom, instruct not to flush when finished. *Comments:*	☐	☐	☐	
32. When client finished expelling enema, assist to clean perineal area, if needed. *Comments:*	☐	☐	☐	
33. Return client to comfortable position. Place clean, dry protective pad under client to catch any solution or feces that may continue to be expelled. *Comments:*	☐	☐	☐	
34. Observe feces and document data. *Comments:*	☐	☐	☐	
35. Remove gloves; wash hands/hand hygiene. *Comments:*	☐	☐	☐	
Return-Flow Enema 36. Wash hands/hand hygiene. *Comments:*	☐	☐	☐	
37. Assess if client understands procedure. *Comments:*	☐	☐	☐	

continued on the following page

continued from the previous page

Procedure 39-7 Administering an Enema	Able to Perform	Able to Perform with Assistance	Unable to Perform	Initials/Date
38. Apply gloves. *Comments:*	☐	☐	☐	
39. Place absorbent pad on bed under client. Assist client into left lateral position with right leg sharply flexed. *Comments:*	☐	☐	☐	
40. If specified, heat solution to desired temperature using thermometer to measure. Solution should be at least body temperature to prevent cramping and discomfort. *Comments:*	☐	☐	☐	
41. Pour solution into bag or bucket, open clamp, and allow solution to prime tubing. Clamp tubing when primed. *Comments:*	☐	☐	☐	
42. Lubricate 5 cm of rectal tube, unless tube is prelubricated. *Comments:*	☐	☐	☐	
43. Holding enema container level with rectum, have client take a deep breath. Simultaneously, slowly and smoothly insert rectal tube into rectum approximately 7–10 cm in an adult. Aim rectal tube toward the client's umbilicus. *Comments:*	☐	☐	☐	

continued on the following page

continued from the previous page

Procedure 39-7 Administering an Enema	Able to Perform	Able to Perform with Assistance	Unable to Perform	Initials/Date
44. Raise container holding solution and open clamp. Solution should be 30–45 cm (12–18 inches) above rectum for an adult. *Comments:*	☐	☐	☐	
45. Slowly administer approximately 200 cc of solution. *Comments:*	☐	☐	☐	
46. Clamp tubing and lower enema container 12–18 inches below client's rectum. Open clamp. *Comments:*	☐	☐	☐	
47. Observe solution container for air bubbles as solution returns. Note any fecal particles. *Comments:*	☐	☐	☐	
48. When no further solution is returned, clamp tubing and raise enema container 12–18 inches above client's rectum. Open clamp, instill approximately 200 cc of fluid. *Comments:*	☐	☐	☐	
49. Repeat raising and lowering solution container until no further flatus is seen. A good rule of thumb is not more than 3 times. *Comments:*	☐	☐	☐	
50. After final return of fluid, clamp tubing and gently remove it from client's anus. Clean anus with tissue to remove any lubricant or solution. *Comments:*	☐	☐	☐	

continued on the following page

continued from the previous page

Procedure 39-7 Administering an Enema	Able to Perform	Able to Perform with Assistance	Unable to Perform	Initials/Date
51. If client feels need to empty rectum, assist onto bedpan or up to bathroom or commode. *Comments:*	☐	☐	☐	
52. When client finished expelling any retained solution, assist to clean perineal area, if needed. *Comments:*	☐	☐	☐	
53. Return client to comfortable position. Place clean, dry protective pad under client. *Comments:*	☐	☐	☐	
54. Observe any expelled solution and document results. *Comments:*	☐	☐	☐	
55. Remove gloves; wash hands/hand hygiene. *Comments:*	☐	☐	☐	

Checklist for Procedure 39-8   Irrigating and Cleaning a Stoma

Name _____ Date _____

School _____

Instructor _____

Course _____

Procedure 39-8 Irrigating and Cleaning a Stoma	Able to Perform	Able to Perform with Assistance	Unable to Perform	Initials/Date
1. Wash hands/hand hygiene. *Comments:*	☐	☐	☐	
2. Apply clean gloves. *Comments:*	☐	☐	☐	
3. Assemble irrigation kit. Attach cone or catheter to irrigation bag tubing. *Comments:*	☐	☐	☐	
4. Fill irrigation bag with 1,000 cc tepid tap water. *Comments:*	☐	☐	☐	
5. Open clamp and let water from irrigation bag fill tubing. *Comments:*	☐	☐	☐	
6. Hang bottom of irrigation bag at height of client's shoulder, or 18 inches above stoma, if client supine. *Comments:*	☐	☐	☐	
7. Check direction of intestine by inserting a gloved finger into orifice of stoma. *Comments:*	☐	☐	☐	
8. Place irrigation sleeve over stoma; hold in place with belt. *Comments:*	☐	☐	☐	

continued on the following page

continued from the previous page

Procedure 39-8 Irrigating and Cleaning a Stoma	Able to Perform	Able to Perform with Assistance	Unable to Perform	Initials/Date
9. Spray inside of irrigation sleeve and bathroom with odor eliminator. *Comments:*	☐	☐	☐	
10. Cuff end of irrigation sleeve and place into toilet bowl or bedpan. *Comments:*	☐	☐	☐	
11. Lubricate cone end of irrigation tubing and insert into stoma orifice through top opening of irrigation sleeve. *Comments:*	☐	☐	☐	
12. Close top of irrigation sleeve over tubing. *Comments:*	☐	☐	☐	
13. Slowly run water through tubing into colon. *Comments:*	☐	☐	☐	
14. Remove cone after all water has emptied out of irrigation bag. *Comments:*	☐	☐	☐	
15. Close end of irrigation sleeve by attaching it to top of sleeve. *Comments:*	☐	☐	☐	
16. Encourage client to ambulate to facilitate emptying remaining stool from colon. *Comments:*	☐	☐	☐	

continued on the following page

continued from the previous page

Procedure 39-8 Irrigating and Cleaning a Stoma	Able to Perform	Able to Perform with Assistance	Unable to Perform	Initials/Date
17. Remove irrigation sleeve after 20–30 minutes or when stool is no longer emptying from colon. *Comments:*	☐	☐	☐	
18. Cleanse stoma and skin with warm tap water. Pat dry. *Comments:*	☐	☐	☐	
19. Place gauze pad over stoma to absorb mucus from stoma. *Comments:*	☐	☐	☐	
20. Secure gauze with hypoallergenic tape. *Comments:*	☐	☐	☐	
21. Remove gloves; wash hands/hand hygiene. *Comments:*	☐	☐	☐	

Checklist for Procedure 40-1   Postoperative Exercise Instruction

Name _____ Date _____

School _____

Instructor _____

Course _____

Procedure 40-1 Postoperative Exercise Instruction	Able to Perform	Able to Perform with Assistance	Unable to Perform	Initials/Date
1. Wash hands/hand hygiene: organize equipment. *Comments:*	☐	☐	☐	
2. Check client's identification band. *Comments:*	☐	☐	☐	
3. Place client in sitting position. *Comments:*	☐	☐	☐	
4. Demonstrate deep breathing exercise. *Comments:*	☐	☐	☐	
5. Have client return demonstrate deep breathing: • Place one hand on abdomen during inhalation. • Expand abdomen and rib cage on inspiration. • Inhale slowly and evenly through nose until maximal chest expansion achieved. • Hold breath for 2–3 seconds. • Slowly exhale through mouth until maximal chest contraction achieved. • Repeat exercise 3 or 4 times; allow client to rest. *Comments:*	☐	☐	☐	
6. Demonstrate splinting and coughing. *Comments:*	☐	☐	☐	

continued on the following page

continued from the previous page

Procedure 40-1 Postoperative Exercise Instruction	Able to Perform	Able to Perform with Assistance	Unable to Perform	Initials/Date
7. Don gloves. *Comments:*	☐	☐	☐	
8. Keep client in sitting position, head slightly flexed, shoulders relaxed and slightly forward, and feet supported on floor. *Comments:*	☐	☐	☐	
9. Teach and return demonstrate splinting and coughing. Have client: • Slowly raise head and sniff air. • Bend forward and exhale slowly through pursed lips. • Repeat breathing 2–3 times. • Place a folded pillow against abdomen when ready to cough; grasp pillow against abdomen with clasped hands. • Take deep breath and begin coughing immediately after completing inspiration by bending forward slightly and producing a series of soft, staccato coughs. • Have tissue ready. *Comments:*	☐	☐	☐	
10. Instruct client on use of an incentive spirometer. Have client: • Hold a volume-oriented incentive spirometer upright. • Take a normal breath and exhale, then seal lips tightly around mouthpiece; take slow, deep breath to elevate the balls in plastic tube; hold inspiration for at least 3 seconds. • Simultaneously, client measures amount of inspired air volume on calibrated plastic tube. • Remove mouthpiece, exhale normally. • Take several normal breaths. • Repeat procedure 4–5 times.	☐	☐	☐	

continued on the following page

continued from the previous page

Procedure 40-1 Postoperative Exercise Instruction	Able to Perform	Able to Perform with Assistance	Unable to Perform	Initials/Date
• Cough after incentive effort; repeat Action 9. Have a tissue ready. • Clean mouthpiece under running water and place in clean container. *Comments:*				
11. Explain leg and foot exercises to client. *Comments:*	☐	☐	☐	
12. Instruct client to return demonstrate in bed. Have client: • With heels on bed, push toes of both feet toward foot of bed until calf muscles tighten; then relax feet. Pull toes toward chin, until calf muscles tighten; then relax feet. • With heels on bed, lift and circle both ankles, first to right and then to left; repeat 3 times; relax. • Flex and extend each knee alternatively, sliding foot up along bed; relax. *Comments:*	☐	☐	☐	
13. Show client how to turn in bed and get out of bed. *Comments:*	☐	☐	☐	
14. Instruct client who will have a left-sided abdominal or chest incision to turn to right side of bed and sit up as follows: • Flex knees. • With right hand splint incision with hand or small pillow. • Turn toward right side by pushing with left foot and grasping shoulder of nurse or foot rail with left hand.	☐	☐	☐	

continued on the following page

continued from the previous page

Procedure 40-1 Postoperative Exercise Instruction	Able to Perform	Able to Perform with Assistance	Unable to Perform	Initials/Date
• Raise up to sitting position on side of bed by using left arm and hand to push down against mattress. *Comments:*				
15. Reverse instructions (use left side instead of right) for client with a right-sided incision according to Action 14. *Comments:*	☐	☐	☐	
16. Instruct clients recovering from orthopedic surgery how to use a trapeze bar. *Comments:*	☐	☐	☐	

Checklist for Procedure 40-2   Pulse Oximetry

Name _____ Date _____

School _____

Instructor _____

Course _____

Procedure 40-2 Pulse Oximetry	Able to Perform	Able to Perform with Assistance	Unable to Perform	Initials/Date
1. Wash hands/hand hygiene. *Comments:*	☐	☐	☐	
2. Select an appropriate sensor, usually fingertip. *Comments:*	☐	☐	☐	
3. Select an appropriate site for sensor. Assess for capillary refill and proximal pulse. *Comments:*	☐	☐	☐	
4. Clean site with alcohol wipe. Remove artificial nails or nail polish, if present, or select another site. Clean any tape adhesive. Use soap and water, if necessary, to clean site. *Comments:*	☐	☐	☐	
5. Apply sensor. Make sure detectors are aligned on opposite sides of selected site. *Comments:*	☐	☐	☐	
6. Connect sensor to oximeter with sensor cable. Turn on machine. Keep plugged in. *Comments:*	☐	☐	☐	

continued on the following page

continued from the previous page

Procedure 40-2 Pulse Oximetry	Able to Perform	Able to Perform with Assistance	Unable to Perform	Initials/Date
7. Adjust alarm limits for high and low O_2 saturation levels, according to manufacturer's directions. Adjust volume. *Comments:*	☐	☐	☐	
8. If taking a reading, note results. If continuous monitoring, move site of spring sensors every 2 hours and adhesive sensors every 4 hours. *Comments:*	☐	☐	☐	
9. Cover sensor with a sheet or towel to protect from exposure to bright light. *Comments:*	☐	☐	☐	
10. Notify prescribing practitioner of abnormal results. *Comments:*	☐	☐	☐	
11. Record results of O_2 saturation measurements, according to prescribing practitioner's order or protocol. Document type of sensor used, application site, hemoglobin levels, and assessment of client's skin at sensor site. *Comments:*	☐	☐	☐	